"The perfect companion for those searching for helpful and valuable information on Lyme Disease and all its idiosyncrasies. A holistic perspective for those in the 'Lyme-Fight' interwoven with meaningful messages of faith".

Renee Lukkason, RN, PHN, BS, and mother of teenager with chronic Lyme Disease

"Cynthia has given us a very special gift to guide us along on our Lyme journey. Her book is powerful but at the same time soothing and encouraging. She offers us a compassionate model for healing."

Neen Lillquist BSN, RN, MNA

"As someone recently diagnosed with Lyme, the information provided in this handbook has been a blessing in helping me better understand Lyme- and what I, and people around me, go through during the treatment. Cynthia's background in medicine, and having been a Lyme sufferer, gives her a depth of knowledge and compassion which she shares in this book to help those dealing with the new epidemic of Lyme."

Bradley Petersen, Outdoor Enthusiast, Photographer

"...Insightful, practical solutions for daily survival- for families, caregivers, and those suffering from symptoms of Chronic Lyme and tick borne diseases. Cynthia, gleaning from her own personal experience, addresses the whole person and is able to offer hope for recovery."

Catherine Morud RNCNP"

"This re-source truly is. For it is a source of knowledge, wisdom, and encouragement that you will re-turn to again and again. Cynthia's personal experience as a sufferer, as well as her nursing expertise, communicate a surprisingly deep and true passion for your wholeness and healing, and will make this handbook a true resource for you and your loved ones."

Isaac Unseth, Pastor of Children's Ministries, Lyme Disease Fighter

Practical Care Tips

For those in the

LYME FIGHT

10.26.13

Dan—

Praying there will be something of help & encouragement for you in this handbook as you battle Lyme—!

Feel free to contact me if you have any questions or are in need of more resources—I'll try to help if I can—

Your Lyme-battle-buddy,

Cynthia Dewhsey

(friend of the famous Paul Nye) ☺

Practical Care Tips

For those in the

LYME FIGHT

An Interactive Care Handbook for

Those Battling Lyme Disease

and Other Chronic Conditions

With Special Notes to Caregivers

Cynthia Dainsberg RN, FCN

BioMed Publishing Group

P.O. Box 550531

South Lake Tahoe, CA 96155

www.LymeBook.com

Copyright 2013 by Cynthia Dainsberg

ISBN: 978-0-9882437-2-9

For related books and DVDs, visit us online at www.LymeBook.com.

DISCLAIMER

This book is not intended as medical advice. It is also not intended to prevent, diagnose, treat or cure disease. Instead, the book is intended only to share the unofficial research and opinion of the author. The book is provided for informational and educational purposes only, not as treatment instructions for any disease. Much of the book is a statement of opinion in areas where the facts are controversial or do not exist. The information in this book should not be considered any more valid than any other type of informal opinion.

The book was not written to replace the advice or care of a qualified health care professional. Be sure to check with your own qualified health care provider before beginning any protocols or procedures discussed in this book, or before stopping or altering any diet, lifestyle, or other therapies previously recommended to you by your health care provider. The treatments described in this book may have side effects and carry other known and unknown risks and health hazards.

Lyme disease is a controversial topic and this book should not be seen as the final word regarding Lyme disease medical care. The statements in this book have not been evaluated by the United States FDA.

Dedicated to Jehovah Jireh

Note that font size and spacing used in this book is intentional to promote the ease of reading this material for persons experiencing 'brain fog', particularly for my 'war buddies' fighting Lyme Disease.

The margins and spaces may be used to jot down your personal notes.

This book is intended to be interactive. You will make the best use of it by: highlighting, jotting notes, making comments, placing the date next to your information with note as to if it was effective, jot down any way you personalize the information… (Perhaps a caregiver or friend can help you make notations if you are unable to do so at this time.)

This book is just a frame-work of ideas to help you establish your own health management plan.

My hope is that it will be a launching pad for you to discover helpful ways to feel the best you can as you battle for optimal health.

Permission given to copy pages for personal use only.

Sections

Acknowledgements

Gratitude most of all- to my Great Physician and Healer - the Lord Jesus Christ.

Thank you for the prayers, support, critiques, and sharing your expertise with me in this project:

My primary Care-Giver, my faithful husband- John, who has been there when I needed him. My children: Casey- my trooper; Christy- my listener; Hunter- my 'tell'. Paul- my dad, who is such a great example of strength and vigor to me. Andrew- my nephew editorial- helper extraordinaire.

Mary V.D.W- my encouraging and inspirational FCN and fb buddy. June, Neen, Renee, James, Kenzie, Gene, Joni, Cathy, CF, Isaac, Brad- and many other fellow Lyme Fighters who support and inspire me....

To Harold and Jeanette, for being so generous with their resource by lending me their healing tool. Bernie and Shirley for providing me with a vital medicinal ingredient ;) Sally- for her foot-washing ministry and for helping make this book possible. And Linda- my walking partner.

Calvary Church- my church family who has been faithful to pray for, and minster to me- the Joy Sisters, Prayer Shawl Ministers, Ladies Day

Out ladies, Elders, Wednesday Night Prayer Team, the men in John's Bible Study group, the 'Lasagna Lady'- Mary, family pizza provider-Ruth, Kathy- prayer support and encouragement... My Stephen's Minster- who has been so faithful to walk this path alongside me, praying for me, and encouraging me each step of the way...

And, the many others who have sent a card, stationary, a plant, quilts; made phone calls, visits, meals... PRAYERS! Special thanks to my doctor- who I'm sure has saved my life!

1. Introduction

I HAVE FOUND *a limited number of resources for those fighting Lyme Disease, that deal with the practical issues of helping to go through the healing process.*

For those who are going through it, the 'healing process' often means: 'worse before better', and that is often an understatement!

Although this is not an exhaustive resource, my hope is that you will find ideas that may ease your day, even a moment, as you fight all those beasties that have been messing with you.

Be encouraged! To you who are fighting this battle, let me say- "You are amazing!" I understand what courage, strength, and fortitude it is taking to hang in there!

For those of you who have picked this up for ideas as a caregiver, let me say- "You are amazing!" It is such a blessing to a Lyme-Fighter to have someone that is not only there for them, but is willing to enter into the fight with them, to encourage and care!

Blessing to all~
Cynthia

2. My Story (part A)

I HAVE AN educational background in health care, and worked for a number of years as an RN before becoming chronically ill from Epstein Barr Virus (EBV), and being diagnosed with Chronic Fatigue Syndrome in 1986 (also known at ME- Myalgic Encephalomyelitis). I had worked in units that included Prolonged Respiratory Care, and a Post-Surgical Step-Down ICU, as well as working in a Blood Center (on and off-site), and in the aphaeresis department.

Another health challenge occurred in 2000, when a vehicle T-boned me. As I was driving north, a vehicle heading east literally flew through a stop sign and impacted my car, directly behind my driver's seat." (Thankfully no one else was in the car with me at the time!) The other driver was driving without a license, and was possibly driving while impaired; he ran from the scene.

I sustained a severe neck sprain, a concussion, and showed signs of internal bleeding. It was a literal blow to my optimal health overall.

Now, besides dealing with the effects of the EBV/CFS/ME, I was also dealing with the effects of having had a concussion and neck sprain; less memory, trouble swallowing, less comfortable positions, and more pain. Eventually I began to experience fibromyalgia like symptoms.

Somewhere along the line, Lyme Disease, with Co-Infections, had entered my body and begun to wreak their havoc as well. For awhile, I just thought the EBV, MVA, and getting older were just all catching up with me! I began to experience new and more intense symptoms; without any real answers from the medical professionals I went to; so I just kept going about life the best I could.

···

In January of 2010, my mom suffered a stroke while at her home in Florida. I flew down with my son to try to be of support, even though I had little reserve myself. Soon after our arrival, my dad took us out for a bite to eat. Though not very hungry due to the shock of everything going on with my mom, we did eat a light fast food meal just because we knew we'd need the energy.

The next day, my dad became extremely ill- to a point that I needed to bring him to the Emergency Room for fluids- he was diagnosed with Norwalk Virus. Come to find out, there was a pandemic going on around us!

My dad was able to come back home later that day, and by late that evening I was going downhill fast! I called my husband back home and told him I just didn't have the strength to help out, and that I felt ill now as well. I became very ill, and my poor dad now had to drive me to the ER!

By the time I got there, I not only was battling Norwalk Virus, very low serum potassium, tachycardia- but I was also experiencing a life-threatening Thyroid Storm.

I was kept in the hospital about three days on IV fluids and meds, and with cardiac monitoring. While hospitalized, my son came down with the Norwalk Virus as well. But thankfully, even while taking care of himself and my dad, my son recovered on his own.

My husband had caught a plane to be with us as soon as he could- finding me in the hospital, our son recovering; and the night he arrived, my dad had another episode for which my husband had to call an ambulance. It turns out my dad had developed C. Diff (Clostridium Difficile) on top of everything else. *I am so thankful my husband listened to me, trusted me, and came as soon as he could!*

So for a time, all three of us were hospitalized- my mom (still in ICU), my dad, and me.

Somehow, I kept trying to do what needed to be done to help my family- but it took everything I had to keep going.

...

My condition worsened physically, emotionally, mentally…and I began to go back to doctors…trying to find someone that

    a.   *wouldn't be* dismissive

    b.   *wouldn't* flatly offer me an anti-depressant

    c.   would be willing to dig in diagnostically!

...

The main point, and of greatest concern to me- was the endocrine symptoms I was having, as well as the tachycardia. I was sent to another endocrinologist- with a TSH of around 9 and flatly told 'nothing was wrong'. I was in such disbelief, so disappointed, feeling so ill- I just wanted to bawl.

I was desperately trying to keep my composure, when the doctor offered me an anti-depressant! (I think it was mostly to make *him* feel better!)

That galled me just enough to make it out of that office to have my cry in the vehicle. My husband had come with me, and was also disappointed that once again- no answers.

More time, more energy, more money- but no answers, and I continued to feel worse and worse.

...

I finally found an Internist who was a good diagnostician, and who had a good understanding of my pre-existing conditions; although I didn't seek him out for it- turns out he is a Lyme Literate Physician. *God was leading me!*

At the end of my appointment, he suggested I may have Lyme Disease. I chuckled to myself- after all, I didn't have any 'bulls-eye' rash or anything... That's a new one, I thought.

But, the doctor asked if I'd ever been tested for it. I hadn't, so my husband and I said 'why not', after all- at least the doctor took me seriously, and he was willing to investigate! So, tests were added to include tests by IGeneX for Lyme, specifically borrelia.

To our amazement, I had positive bands show up indicating Lyme was at play.

In July of 2011, I began treatment for Late Stage Lyme- Neuroborreliosis, and a number of Co-Infections (erhlichia, Anaplasma, Rickettsia, Babesia, Bartonella). The infections were affecting my brain, endocrine system, muscles, digestive tract, heart, eyes....

Within two weeks I had my first two "Herx-like" reactions. (Basically, the term 'Herx' come from Herxheimer Reactions- named after a doctor who first observed the severe reactions patients had when treated for spirochete infections).

These reactions can be very severe- even to the point of death, if not handled carefully. At the least- you feel like a 'Mack Truck ran you over'. Basically, any and all symptoms you've been having show up with great intensity, almost all at once.

The Herx reaction is thought to occur because of your body systems being overwhelmed by the organism debris from the treatment killing them off; not only does the debris overwhelm your systems (blood, kidney, liver, respiratory, muscular…), but the debris is thought to be toxic! And, neurotoxins adversely affect brain function.

Others believe that as the organisms are attacked, this stirs our cytokines (WBC) to bring about an overwhelming response, causing us to feel so ill.

Either way, rotten does not even begin to describe how intensely ill you can become.

...

HINT: *There are some people who have Lyme Disease that for some reason do not Herx. So although it is a hallmark of sorts for many, just because someone doesn't Herx, doesn't mean they don't have Lyme, or that the treatment isn't working. If this is your case- be sure to check with your physician about it.*

...

The second Herx came on the second week of treatment; feeling quite ill, it sent me to the ER due to the pressure in my chest and trouble breathing. I'd never experienced such fear and dread as I did during that Herx!

That was my welcome into the world of Late-Stage Lyme Disease.

The first 6+ months of treatments held only a handful of bright spots; most of those months were spent living life horizontally- in bed, on a couch, even on the floor.

There were times when I'd start to feel up to being about, maybe get out of the house a couple hours, but then I'd spend days trying to recover.

For those who know how the flu feels- imagine those symptoms greatly magnified and going on for months, with some wax-n-waning...

•••

Not only was I a mess physically, but emotionally and mentally as well. The infections played havoc with my emotions by attacking my brain and endocrine system, not to mention all the other challenges you have when ill a long time.

Mentally it was tough because not only was the infection in my brain- but when the treatments were working and killing off the organisms- it would leave me with extreme fogginess, forgetfulness, irritability, hyper-sensitivity, emotionally labile, headaches, aches and pains...

That's when I came to learn about detoxifying techniques like the foot soaks, baths, lemon in water, juicing...

•••

To be continued...

3. The Art of Therapeutic Baths to detoxify from the treatments, and for comfort

My Own Journey into the 'Art of a Bath'

When I hear the word *bath*, images and stories come to my mind.

As a small child, I remember my mother giving me a bath in the kitchen sink, and later-the joy of a tub-bath. The tub-bath was especially wonderful when I'd have just enough water to create spectacular waves;

the trickiest part was to do this while still maintaining as much dry ground around the tub as possible (as parents don't seem to have the same appreciation for these aquatic feats if water is found dripping from the ceiling in the room below)!

As a youth, we didn't have an air conditioner to cool us off after a hot summer day. However, I fondly remember many a pleasant, warm summer evening, taking a dip in the lake for a cooling bath before heading to bed.

My dad has told us his own 'bathing stories' from his stint as an Army soldier overseas during World War II:

> *"While at Cirey, France we hadn't had a bath or shower for over a month! The nuns in town had a public bath that they ran; one night we all went over there in shifts- man did that feel good!!!!*

I had been feeling OK but after the bath and "shedding" all of the dirt I ended up with a bad cold."

Speaking of baths overseas, although I didn't actually take a bath in the Bath Houses, I have fond memories of a trip to the British Isles with my mom- during which we visited the ancient city of Bath. Here, Romans brought bathing to the Isles in a *big* way.

●●●

Recently, while herxing and having been very isolated from people outside of my family- I had carefully made my way out onto our front porch, to take in the fresh air, and enjoy a shaded spot from which to look out onto the sun-drenched pasture about me.

Everything ached, including my feet. I was so fatigued. I couldn't even muster enough strength and energy to self-massage my feet.

My family happened to have all been gone at the time, so I had no one to ask to massage my feet. Not to mention, I didn't want to bother my family with *another* request anyway, as they were already burdened with extra duties.

Still- *oh* how my feet ached, and *oh* how I wanted a foot massage.

●●●

I was sitting there feeling quite pathetic and alone. In my heart I cried out to God about my misery, about how alone I felt; tears fell.

I just felt so ill, so tired, so weak… Only God knew how I was feeling, and how badly I wanted a foot massage… and that would have to be good enough.

●●●

In a little while, a friend of mine from church drove up unexpectedly. I was glad to see her, but still had no idea *how* glad I would be.

Curiously, she had a basin in one hand and, and a handbag in the other; she told me to stay seated out on the porch, and 'may (she) just go into the house for something and come right back out?'

"Sure", I said, not having much energy to refuse, and being quite curious about what she was up to.

She came out shortly with the basin now filled with hot water, or rather-water that was the *perfect* temperature!

She gently set my already bare feet into the basin, and immediately my feet began to be soothed.

My friend sat there on the porch floor in front of me and chatted with me.

New tears flowed from my eyes- this was a very humbling experience. To be served this way- truly she was God-sent to me.

After having my feet soaked, one-by-one she gently massaged each foot with oil. What heavenly relief!

I am now convinced that whether it's a full bath, or a foot bath, the whole process is beneficial. So I began my journey into baths to detoxify and heal.

...

Whether you have always been a 'bath person', or not- I hope you find something of benefit to you in these pages.

Perhaps, like me, you have been 'forced' into becoming a bath person- in which case, I especially hope you'll find that these ideas help to bring about better days for you.

Inside Out

A therapeutic bath first begins by making sure you are well hydrated before, during, and after your bath. (Yes, even if only doing a foot bath.)

...

Hydration is very important to promoting optimal health, and to help your body eliminate toxins and waste effectively. Water is a valuable agent in helping you move toxins out of your body.

Make sure you are getting an adequate intake of water on a daily basis, 6-8 glasses of water a day is a good start; or figure on drinking 1/2 your body weight in ounces.

Remember that beverages containing caffeine *do not* hydrate, they promote dehydration.

Also, beware of sugar laden drinks, as sugar promotes unwanted inflammation (not to mention it can make the beasties thrive)!

Beware of alcoholic beverages, which will adversely affect your body's ability to filter out toxins, as well as there being potentially dangerous affects when one drinks alcohol while taking a hot bath.

...

You may want to check into taking a high-quality Chlorella product to facilitate removing toxins. It can come in liquid or capsules. Make sure it is a pure product and is proven to be well absorbed. If your body has a difficult time removing toxins- you may ask your physician about taking Cholestyramine™.

...

When taking detoxifying baths- it is good to drink water (or another healthy drink) before, during and after your bath.

•••

HINT: *Yes, you will want to make sure to empty your bladder before you begin, and after, you take your bath!*

•••

If you would like to spruce up your water- try adding fresh lemon or grapefruit juice, or perhaps a sprig of mint. *Be aware, if you do add lemon juice to your water- use a straw to drink from it, as lemon juice can be harming to tooth enamel.*

If you are very hardy - you may try a glass of water in which you add a teaspoon of Apple Cider Vinegar (ACV), and a teaspoon of blackstrap molasses. (Bragg's ™ brand of ACV is excellent.)

HINT: *Anecdote for the ladies: I had night-sweats for over 20 years- they eventually faded away the further along I got into treatments for Lyme; then I was overcome with 'hot flashes'.*

The flashes would hit me about 9pm, waking me up many times during the night (like you need your sleep interrupted any more than it already is), and then abate about 6am. In my search for a 'fun-something-to-drink' with my evening snack- I took to mixing up ACV, molasses in a glass of cold water.

After a few days, I was amazed to find the hot flashes were gone! I looked it up on the internet, and found others had gotten relief from hot flashes with that concoction as well! I still don't know what the action of it is- the amino acids, vitamins or minerals... All I know is that I will be sticking with it for my evening beverage!

•••

Another refreshing beverage you can mix up is 1 cup water, 1 teaspoon ACV, 1 teaspoon Stevia™, and 1 tablespoon fresh gingerroot (remove skin, and finely chopped root). Put into glass container, like a canning jar, cover and refrigerate. (Or, mix 8 cups cold water, 12 teaspoons Stevia™, 1/3 cup ACV, 1 teaspoon gingerroot powder. Keep refrigerated.)

•••

If your favorite beverage is a cup of decaffeinated green tea, or herbal tea; hot tea will promote sweating-out toxins too.

To help replace minerals, you may try drinking a vegetable juice drink; like carrot juice, or your favorite vegetable juicing concoction.

Coconut water has healthy benefits as well. You can drink coconut water cold, or you may want to try coconut milk mixed into hot water for a hot drink (I add a single serving of Stevia™ to sweeten it).

HINT: *If you are already taking vitamin C in your daily health regimen, take your tolerated dose before and after your bath. This can help your body send toxins into your blood-stream, and move them closer to where your body can get rid of them during your bath time. Also, if you are taking antioxidant nutritional supplements, plan to take them before and after your bath.*

•••

Skin Care

The largest organ of your body is your skin. It deserves some special attention.

The condition of your skin can give many clues about the status of your health, so while preparing for a bath- you have a wonderful opportunity to make note of any changes in your skin; and alert your Health Care

Provider should you notice any changes of concern.

Be sure to be thoughtful about what you put on your skin. Pay attention to the materials you wear, as well as any lotions or oils that you apply.

Be most cautious about using those things which contain materials that are synthetically/chemically produced. Natural material and ingredients will be most friendly to your skin. (Be careful of natural ingredients to which you may be allergic.)

Everyone's skin handles sun exposure differently. Take caution against sustaining sun burns. Try to stay out of the sun when it is at its peak for UV rays (like from 11am-2pm). Be aware of any of your medications which caution you about being out in the sun.

If you must be in the sun, try wearing light clothing which blocks UV rays. Wear a hat that not only shields your face, but also make sure your ears and neck are protected.

If you feel you must apply a 'sun protection lotion', be sure to read the ingredients and use lists carefully.

Remember too that there are supplements that are thought to help protect you against sunburn, such as the supplement Astaxanthin.

Did you know that our outer skin was created to have an invisible germ protecting barrier? It is called the acid mantle.

This acid mantle discourages bacteria and viruses from taking hold of you. As its name implies, in proper balance, the optimal pH of this acid mantle should be 5.5 on the pH scale.

As you may recall from high school, a pH of 7 is neutral, lower is acidic, higher is alkaline.

HINT: *If you are using any soap products or ingredients such as baking soda, which is very alkaline (pH 8.2),*

you may want to top-off your bath by adding apple cider vinegar to the water; or, some may prefer to apply coconut oil after their bath, as coconut is acidic in nature- either can help restore your acid mantle pH.

(Perhaps my dad, and his Army buddies, would've done well to have known this!)

■■■

HINT: *Sea Salt is generally neutral, and Epsom Salt ranges from 5.5-6.5.*

■■■

You may want to add 'skin brushing' to your bathing routine to enhance the benefit of detoxifying.

Your skin is a very important organ for detoxification, along with your lungs, kidneys, liver and colon.

Your feet can be an especially good place from which toxins can be released.

■■■

Skin brushing is done before your bath, while your skin is dry.

You will want to use a brush made with natural bristles. Begin with your feet, and move upwards and inwards.

Don't forget your arms, but *do not brush your face.*

Move the brush in circular motions, and towards the heart, in nice even and gentle strokes.

Many people believe that practicing skin brushing opens the pores of your skin to facilitate detoxification- *and, it feels good!*

General Bathing Guidelines- Including Precautions

First, please **check with your Health Care Provider before beginning these baths**; especially if you have any history of high or low blood pressure, heart or kidney disease, are diabetic, or pregnant, POTS ... or any other health challenges.

Also- if the water you use for bathing is 'city water' (treated)- I encourage you to get a filter for your tub water, so that your body won't be exposed to chlorine byproducts, or other impurities, as you bathe.

...

Once you have gotten the approval to begin- it is always wise to begin slowly.

You will want to start out with fewer ingredients for a shorter amount of time- until you know how you will respond to any of the baths suggested.

Try the basic recipes first. You may even want to have someone with you until you know how well you will tolerate any given bath.

...

NOTE: *If at any time you feel lightheaded, or experience dizziness, headache, exhaustion, fatigue, nausea, or weakness- STOP your bath, and ask for assistance.*

...

You may skin brush, and/or shower prior to your bath to help remove any excess body oils, dead skin or accumulated toxins.

If you shower, use a mild, well tolerated soap, and a rough washcloth or loofa sponge. *Rinse thoroughly.*

•••

Make sure the tub you are using is not only clean, but that any substances used to clean it are removed.

Many cleaning solutions may be toxic, and our objective here is to *de*toxify!

•••

Fill the tub with water that is as hot as you can tolerate, without burning your skin.

The water should be very warm, but no more than 98 degrees F.

The warm water will draw the toxins out of the body to the skin's surface, and as the water begins to cool, the toxins will be pulled out from the skin.

Basically, sweating in the tub is a good thing; sweating is valuable mechanism to release toxins. Later, we will discuss additions to your bath water that will further promote sweating.

•••

There should be enough water in the tub for you to comfortably immerse your body up to your neck.

•••

In keeping with starting out slowly - begin with only a plain-water, five-minute soak for your first bath.

In subsequent baths, increase the time at five-minute intervals as tolerated, until you have reached a 20-30 minute soak without any ill effects.

Keep in mind, part of the reason for starting out with shorter times is that you may feel well enough while in the tub, but you may feel unwell afterward- or even the next day.

So be kind and gentle to your body in this process. Once you have worked up to tolerating a thirty minute, plain water bath, without any ill effects, you may begin detoxifying baths.

•••

For those of you practicing detoxifying bathing during treatments for Lyme Disease- baths can be taken daily (as tolerated) during times you most need to detoxify.

•••

HINT: *Rotate the type of bath you use each day to experience greater effectiveness; unless it is an Epsom Salt bath, which can be taken daily.*

•••

Staying ahead on the detoxifying process by using detoxifying baths can be to your advantage.

Once you are through a particular time of needing to detoxify, then you may choose the kind of bath and frequency that best meets your needs.

Generally, detoxifying baths may be taken three times a week, until your general health has improved.

For maintenance, to keep toxins from accumulating, use the baths once or twice a week.

Keep a loofa sponge handy, or a skin brush approved for water, as you may want to gently massage your skin and muscle areas while in the bath to increase your circulation to the skin.

...

After you have successfully finished your detoxifying bath- it is a good rule-of-thumb to again shower, to cleanse any toxins deposited on your skin from the bath. Wash your hair as well. You do not want to give your body an opportunity to reabsorb any toxins it's kicked out onto the skin!

If you experience further perspiration, or begin again to perspire, you will want to repeat the shower.

...

HINT: *You may want to just wrap yourself up in a warm, absorbent towel... and put on a pair of clean, warm, naturally woven socks and relax in a chair until you think you have finished sweating- then wash off.*

...

You will want to gather your bath items before you begin your bath. On the next page you will find a checklist to help you get started.

Add your own items, depending on which bath recipes you like to use. You may want to copy the Bath Checklist page for your own use.

Bathing Checklist-

☐ Thermometer (can use a kitchen candy-thermometer)

☐ Towels, absorbent (one bath towel, one hand or face towel)

☐ Nonslip bath mat

☐ Measuring tools

☐ Bath recipe ingredients

☐ Timer

☐ Beverage in a non-breakable container

☐ Help, when starting out, or on those weak-days- don't hesitate to ask for help~

☐ Focus material (see page 48 regarding Focus)

☐ Warm, dry socks

☐ Natural bristled skin brush (2 if possible, one for dry brushing, one for in tub)

☐ Soap with natural ingredients

☐ Apple Cider Vinegar (if using any ingredients that may disrupt your skin mantle)

☐ Neck pillow (For this, you may use an old fashioned water bottle filled with warm water.)

☐ Essential oils

☐ Body oil (coconut, almond, sesame… no mineral oil)

☐ OTHER:

HINT: *You may want to keep your checklist and things most often used together in a basket near your bath; restock your basket right after your bath- so you're ready to go for the next bath.*

Recipes

Now that you have worked up from plain bath water, you are ready to try the following recipes; but, where to start?

To begin, here is some beneficial information on the various ingredients you will find in the following recipes to better help you determine which bath you may choose to meet your needs.

...

Epsom Salt: detoxifies, kills parasites, bactericidal, antiviral. The magnesium sulfate in the salt can be absorbed by your skin, which can draw toxins from the body, calm the nervous system, relax muscles, reduce swelling, act as a moisturizer, and remove dead skin cells.

Dead Sea Salt: minerals to soothe and helps to pull out toxins. Only 12-18% salinity of the Dead Sea salt is sodium chloride, it is very high in bromide ions, and it is low in pH. It is unlike ocean sea salt, which is 97% sodium chloride. For more benefits, go to <u>www.health-benefit-of-water.com/sea-salt.html</u>

Apple Cider Vinegar (ACV)- promotes and restores proper skin pH, anti-bacterial, contains amino acids/enzymes

Baking Soda- alkalizing, cleansing (use ACV afterward to restore proper pH of skin mantle)

Hydrogen Peroxide- promotes oxygenation, which can kill bacteria and viruses.

Herbal teas- (see specific herb)

...

HINT: *Stay away from any herbal teas, or oils to which you have sensitivities or allergies.*

...

Essential oils *(with commonly associated benefits noted)*

Copaiba- anti-inflammatory, ant-bacterial, anti-arthritic, soothes digestion

Chamomile- anti oxidant, relaxant, soothing, promotes healthy skin

Eucalyptus– anti-bacterial, antiviral, antifungal, expectorant

Ginger- helps soothes nausea, soothes muscular aches and pains, helps clear respiratory congestion and infection

Grapefruit- metabolic stimulator, cleansing, promotes lymphatic and vascular system, antidepressant, relaxant

Lemon- antiseptic, immune stimulant, improves memory, relaxant

Lemongrass- Purifying, anti-parasitic, anti-inflammatory, improves circulation, promotes lymph flow

Lavender- soporific, calming, relaxant, antiseptic, anti-fungal, combats excess sebum on skin

Nutmeg- anti-inflammatory, antiseptic, anti-parasitic, analgesic, adrenal stimulant, muscle relaxant, increases production of melatonin

Orange-relaxant, circulatory stimulant

Oregano- anti-aging, anti-viral, antibacterial, antifungal, anti-parasitic, anti-inflammatory, immune stimulant

Peppermint-anti-inflammatory, anti-parasitic, anti-bacterial, antiviral, antifungal, digestive stimulant, pain-relieving

Other:

...

Oils: Sesame oil is the only oil which promotes continued detoxification once applied. You may apply it before or after a bath to promote detoxification. It can also be put into your bath water- but *check with your tub manufacturer first.*

Full Bath Recipes

Basic Epsom Salt Bath ~ soothes muscles

Begin with ¼ cup Epsom Salts. You may gradually increase the amount of Epsom Salts with each bath, up to using 4 cups per tub.

Remember to start out slowly, and stop the bath if you experience any symptoms. Work your way up to a 30 minute soak without symptoms.

Lemony Salt Bath ~ soothes nerves, uplifting

1 cup Dead Sea Salt

½ cup fresh lemon

After the Dead Sea Salt is dissolved in the bath water, squeeze the juice of half a lemon into the water, and then the rind.

•••

Dead Sea Salt & Epsom Salt Bath ~ soothing to muscles and skin

½ cup Epsom Salt and ½ cup Dead Sea Salt for every 60 pounds of body weight

•••

Dead Sea Salt, Epsom Salt & Sesame Oil Bath ~ soothing and detoxifying

(Before using this recipe- check with your manufacturer's manual regarding use of any oil in your tub) This recipe is especially helpful to those experiencing dry skin and stress: 1 cup Sea Salt, 1 Cup Epsom Salt, 1 cup Sesame Oil

Soak 20 minutes; pat yourself dry.

Apple Cider Vinegar Bath ~ promotes healthy skin pH

Start by using ¼ cup of *Apple Cider Vinegar*. (*Do not use white vinegar.*)

If tolerated well, you may gradually increase amount with each bath, up to 1 cup per bath.

•••

Hydrogen Peroxide Bath ~ invigorating and promotes oxygenation

Use up to 8 oz of food-grade 35% hydrogen peroxide in a half-full tub of *warm* water.

This particular bath has the potential to increase your alertness, so it is not recommended to do before bedtime.

HINT: *Note also for this bath, you want warm water, not hot. Hot water will cause the hydrogen peroxide to deteriorate too quickly and you won't get maximum benefit.*

HINT: *This bath has the potential to increase oxygen at the cellular level (very good for those fighting Lyme Disease).*

•••

Soda & Dead Sea Salt Bath ~ soothing

This bath can be especially good for detoxifying from X-ray and radiation exposure.

Use equal amounts of baking soda and non-iodized Dead Sea Salt. Slowly build up to one-pound of each.

...

Ginger Root Bath ~ detoxifying and soothing

Option 1: Cut a thumb-size piece of ginger root into small pieces, put these pieces into a small pot of water on the stove, bring to a boil. Steep, with heat off, for 30 minutes. Strain out the particles; pour the *liquid* into a full bath.

Option 2: In a small bowl of water, stir in one cup of Epsom Salts, and 2 tablespoons of ginger powder. Once mixed, add this to a full tub of water. It is recommended that you do not exceed 30 minutes in this bath solution.

Option 3: Freshly grate 2 Tablespoons of ginger root and place it into a tea-ball; place this in your bath water.

...

Herbal Tea Bath customize to suit your need

Use one cup of brewed tea in a full tub. If you are sensitive to any of these herbs, you may not tolerate them in a bath. Also, *do not* use more than one kind of tea in a bath at a time.

(Some recommended teas to try are: Catnip, Yarrow, Peppermint, Pleurisy root, Chamomile, Vervain, Horsetail)

Essential Oils - Customize to suit your need

Use the basic recipe for Epsom Salts and add you favorite essential oil. Make sure that you are using a pure, high quality brand essential oil.

• • •

HINT: *Although essential oils have aromatic value- for thousands of years, these oils have been highly valued medicinally.*

• • •

HINT: *Avoid the oils of any scents to which you are allergic. And do* not *use them while pregnant without first consulting your physician.*

• • •

Some specific oils and their potential benefits are listed on pages 23-24.

• • •

Note of caution: check your manufacturing information to make sure if oils can be used in your tub. Most recommend that oils *not* be used when running jets.

HINT: *As you try each Bath Recipe, make your own notations here, or next to the recipe. You may put things like the date you tried it, how well you tolerated it, how long you bathed, give it a 1-5 star rating, make any* *notes on how you personalized it… You may also want to update and further personalize your Bath Checklist.*

Notes:

...

Foot Baths

Foot baths are very therapeutic as well; they have the advantages of being economical, and portable- which is a great option for those without a bath tub available.

(I like to sit out on our porch in the summer and soak my feet; or perhaps you want to bless someone else by going to their house to treat them to a foot bath).

The bottoms of your feet have some of the largest pores of your body- which makes a foot bath a great option for detoxifying.

You may apply some of the principles of full bath guidelines to your Foot Baths, such as: water temperature, soaking time, skin preparation with dry brushing, drink fluids before, during and after…

Also, following your foot bath, you may want to gently scrub your feet with a loofa sponge or natural fiber brush.

Gel, or lotion, of 100% Aloe Vera can be used to moisturize your feet after your foot bath. Other lotions may have fragrances, chemicals, dyes, etc; which you do not want to be reabsorbed by your feet.

Foot baths can be done daily as needed, and about once a week for maintenance if being used for detoxifying.

■■■

You will need to have a container in which your feet fit comfortably, the water level can safely be well up into calf area, and be able to withstand very warm/hot water.

Make sure all of your supplies are within reach, and that you have whatever supplies you need for after your soak.

■■■

HINT: *You may want to make a personal copy of the Bath Checklist to use for Foot Baths as well. Add anything specific you need to personalize it; like the Foot Bath tub, a bath matt to place under the tub…*

Recipe A

General Foot Bath

Basic, to sooth muscles and detox

Mix together: 1 cup Dead Sea Salt, 1 cup of Epsom Salts, 2 cups of baking soda. Store mix in an airtight container (preferably glass).

Option: add 4-6 drops of your favorite essential oil

Use about ¼ cup of mix per foot bath.

...

Recipe B

Ginger-Snap-Foot Bath

Cleansing, uplifting, soothing, stimulating

Mix 1 cup Epsom Salts with 2 Tablespoons of ginger root powder, then add to your foot bath water.

...

Recipe C

Two-Teas Foot Rescue Bath
Soothing and purifying

To your foot bath, add 1 cup Epsom Salts and one bag each of peppermint tea and chamomile tea.

Let these 'steep' for about 10 minutes.

Remove the tea bags, and then you may soak for about 30 minutes.

This recipe can be especially soothing and relaxing, as well as detoxifying and deodorizing.

...

Recipe D

Honey-Sweet Feet Foot Bath
Anti-bacterial, soothing, cleansing

Mix into your foot bath:

1 Tablespoon of honey

1 Tablespoon of natural, gentle liquid soap

1 teaspoon of pure vanilla extract

2 Tablespoons of sweet almond oil

Honey has antibacterial and antifungal properties. Honey can also act as an antioxidant, exfoliator and moisturizer; meanwhile, the oils can help soften rough skin.

...

Recipe E

Parsley, Tea & Me Foot Bath
Cleansing, soothing

Steep these ingredients per one gallon of hot water for 10 minutes, before soaking your feet:

4 bags of chamomile tea

1/8 cup dried parsley

4 drops of essential oil of your choice

...

Recipe F

Salty Dog Foot Bath

soothing and detoxifying

Mix 2 cups Kosher Salt with 1 cup Epsom Salts.

Optional addition: 4 drops of your choice essential oil

...

Recipe G

"Hot Stuff" Foot Bath

Promotes sweating to augment detoxifying, increase circulation, pain relief...

To your foot bath water, add:

1 Tablespoon of Mustard Powder and 1 teaspoon of Cayenne Powder

This combination will help raise your core body temp.

...

HINT: *To make your foot bath even more soothing- you may place several small marbles, floral round glass marbles, or smooth river rocks to the bottom of your foot bath basin. Gently move your feet over them while you are soaking.*

...

My Favorite Baths	Date of Bath

The Art of Relaxation and Rejuvenation

Clear Focus

For anyone who has been through childbirth, or any other traumatic and painful event - you know how important 'focus' can be when you are overwhelmed, especially by pain and anxiety.

In those moments it can be a huge help to have that One Thing, or One Person, on which to focus, to help you get through it, and to help calm the storm.

It will be something or someone… different for each person. And, you may even have a different focus object for different challenges you are facing.

The important thing is that you think through what it is that will help you the most to focus on; what thing, or person, will be a good distraction for you.

A good distraction will be something that not only will take your mind away from the discomfort, not to escape it, but rather to help you to go *through* it; something that will bring *you strength, courage, and peace.*

...

I call them 'love handles'- to help me handle the situation, something I can hold onto! For me- it is most usually, the LORD.

In the middle of the worst Herx I've had (sent me to ER)- the pain, discomfort and anxiety where overwhelming. My head was spinning, my heart was pounding, my body was writhing…

I was desperate to breathe! My chest felt as if it were being crushed, I felt like I was going to die. I was deeply afraid! Nothing felt safe or secure! I had been praying for relief from the symptoms- but they only seemed to mount.

Finally- in my soul, I cried out to God and told Him I was afraid, that I needed something to hold on to! I felt like *everything* was unstable!

He answered with an amazing sense of calm and whispered to my soul that He Himself is my Safe Place.

He reminded me that He was with me, no matter the circumstances, no matter how I was feeling- being with Him, I felt safe.

I didn't focus on safety or peace- *but by focusing on Him, He gave me safety and peace.*

Experiencing dread, anxiousness, panic—any of these are hard to 'override' even with our best effort, and trying different techniques. But the focus can help you ride it out. *For me through, I've found that in focusing on the LORD: He is the only One that can over-ride those times.*

•••

Whatever you decide on for your focus, do keep it simple- as you know, when those tough times come- there isn't a lot of cognitive energy to use.

On what, or who, can you focus to help you? *(Note which focus has helped, and under which circumstance or with what feelings... For some- it may be a person, or a place, a picture, a song, a word...)*

...

Beauty

This is a good place to bring up Beauty. Perhaps your choice of focus will be an object of beauty.

I remember how during the worst of times in my illness- the world seemed to go into a grey-scale.

It would help so much to find even a singular thing of beauty at which to look- to soak in. A picture of a beautiful place, a beautiful object, even color alone can have benefit- inspiring beauty.

Colors can bring joy and comfort to your senses. You can add color to your day by:

Getting some colored pillow cases

■■■

Put a green plant in your room

■■■

Colored sheets or throw

■■■

Pajamas in cheery colors

■■■

Add a full-spectrum light (such as an OTT light) if light is tolerated

■■■

Consider new window treatments

■■■

Make drinking liquids more fun with colored cups/glasses/mugs

■■■

Add wall art with colors that are therapeutic (inexpensive frames, your own enlarged photos)…

■■■

Different colors tend to give different affects. Besides our having favorite colors- there may be a reason for it.

What colors help you feel: happy, peaceful, warmer, cooler... Here are some ideas to help you choose colors.

HINT: *Remember- even a little bit of color can go a long way.*

Red- can symbolize life, strength, and vitality; be warming, and help reduce anxiety

■ ■ ■

Pink- can symbolize love, warmth

■ ■ ■

Orange- another warm color; stimulating, and can symbolize joy

■ ■ ■

Yellow- a warm color and is thought to be stimulating (use judiciously as it can be over-stimulating as well)

■ ■ ■

Green- is calming, restful and peaceful

■ ■ ■

Blue- calming, cooling, and relaxing. (Stay away from the darker tones though, as they can be more depressive.)

■ ■ ■

Violet- symbolizes dignity and can help calm the nervous system

∎∎∎

Magenta- thought to have a freeing quality; especially helpful in combination with a complimentary green.

∎∎∎

Hint: You can keep a room in neutrals and just add splashes of color to suit your mood, or how you are feeling that day.

Perhaps a friend would be willing to bring you color swatches from a local paint store for you to look over...see which ones you most like, and notice what kind of emotional response, if any, you have to the color (energizing, calming, like it, don't like it). This may help you decide what colors you may want to keep handy for 'those days'.

You may have someone who would be willing to find sheets, or pillow-cases, or window treatments, or pajamas... in colors that add beauty to your day.

∎∎∎

My sister-in-law got me a subscription to a home magazine. Each month the magazine highlights a palette of colors for painting.

When there is a palette that is especially pleasing to me, I tear out the page and tape it to the wall in front of me. Just looking at the colors gives me a lift, and as the sun streams in differently through the day- the colors' hues change as well.

For those of us living in 'small worlds', even this can bring an aspect of enjoyment and beauty into our lives.

Friends of mine gifted me with beautiful quilts and prayer shawls to brighten even my resting times, and soothe the chills...

●●●

If light sensitivity is an issue for you, a sleeping-mask may help to block out light. If certain lights are bothersome, try wearing a brimmed hat; you may even try wearing glasses with different colored lenses. You can start off with trying different sunglasses.

If sunglasses don't help, check online at http://irlen.com/ (Irlen Method) to find out more about how you may choose from a variety of colored lenses that may be of help to you.

If the background colors on your computer bother you- Try using the applications which allow you to change the background color and font size. You can also try out different colored backgrounds at the Irlen Method website.

What kinds of things are beautiful to you?

What colors help you to feel:

Peace-

Joy-

Energized-

Soothed-

Strong-

What ideas do you have to add simple touches of beauty to your recovery-living area?

Breathe

Many of us Lyme Warriors have had air hunger. Deep breathing promotes oxygenation, relaxation, and helps our body clear out toxins. Even those who are healthy can benefit from learning good deep breathing exercises.

●●●

First, be mindful of keeping good posture while standing, or sitting, in particular. I haven't always had the best posture, but I've noticed since being ill I do a lot of 'leaning forward', and I have a tendency to tense up my shoulder & neck muscles. So, I have been working on re-training myself to use better posture.

It's not easy, and I have to frequently remind myself (sticky notes on mirrors), but the benefits are worth it (*even for old dogs like me*).

If your posture could use a tune-up, check yourself in the mirror, see that you retract your shoulders comfortably to help get good alignment and stand as tall as possible.

If you notice you are tense in the shoulder and neck area, gently do a few shoulder-rolls, to the front and then to the back. Only do what is comfortable for you- not too fast, or vigorous.

To do a Shoulder Roll: while standing or sitting with good posture, at the same time, gently move your shoulders in such a way that your moving them in a circular-like fashion to the forward, down, back, up, forward, down…

After a few rolls that direction- do the same type of movement, only in reverse; back, down, forward, up, back, down…

●●●

Now, there are a number of breathing exercises, but I will first go over general proper breathing techniques, and then I will give you one deep breathing exercise.

Proper breathing; it may sound funny to practice proper breathing, but actually, most people do not take proper breaths. To help you learn what proper breathing is, try this exercise while lying down on the floor (if you are able). You may have a rug or blanket under you.

Lie down with your legs straight and your arms at your side (not touching your body) with palms up. You may close your eyes. Take time to just relax your body and breathe freely. (If you cannot lie on the floor- you may sit in a comfortable chair; place one hand on your abdomen and the other on your chest, and follow these instructions.)

Breathe in through your nose, keeping your mouth closed as you breathe.

Notice which, your abdomen or chest, is moving the most; if your chest is doing the work- you are actually only getting shallow breaths. If you are using your abdomen- you are making the best use of your lungs! If breathing properly, you should feel your abdomen rise as you breathe in, and fall as you let breath out. Your chest should only move slightly.

Now that you have a good idea of what a proper breath feels like, be aware throughout the day of how you are breathing- if you catch yourself 'chest-breathing', consciously take a few deep-belly breaths to remind your body of using your lungs well.

Most germs do not do well in oxygenated environments- so the more you are using proper breathing techniques, the more you are helping your body to *not* be a good home to germs!

...

Here is a deep breathing technique you may want to do when you are stressed:

This technique can be done while either lying down as stated, or by sitting up straight in a comfortable chair:

Note: *If at any time you feel dizzy- you are probably breathing to quickly- remember to use slow, steady breaths.*

Lie on your back, on a rug or blanket on the floor. Keep your knees bent, your feet about apart about eight inches, and your toes pointed outward slightly.

Keep your spine nice and straight.

Put one hand on your belly, and one on your chest.

Now, inhale slowly and deeply through your nose. Allow your abdomen to gently push up your hand as far you feel comfortable. (Your chest should only move slightly.)

Continue to breathe in and out this way until it becomes rhythmic and comfortable.

Inhale through your nose and exhale through your mouth (with 'pursed lips')- making a quiet, breeze like sound, as you gently breathe out (as if gently blowing out a candle).

Keep your jaw muscles relaxed. Take long, slow, deep breaths- gently raising and lowering your abdomen.

Beginning this technique, start with doing this for only 5 minutes; as you become more comfortable with it, you may do it for up to 20 minutes.

After your time of deep breathing, stay still for a few minutes and return to your natural regular breathing pattern while allowing your body to remain relaxed.

Write your own goal as to how and when you will practice deep breathing technique:

After you have met your goal of practicing deep breathing techniques- write down any differences you have noticed in how you are feeling, and when have you found it most helpful:

Courage and Strength

Let me just tell you, if you are battling an illness, especially a chronic condition: "You have courage!" Only those who've been in the battle really get it. So, if you've never heard that you are courageous before- hear it now from me!

Many times, even our loved ones are unable to encourage us, we must learn the fine art of self-encouragement. And, just as we don't care for others to use flattery, or vain encouragement- we must not do it to ourselves. Jot in a journal about what accomplishment you've had for the day, even if it's sitting in a chair for 20 minutes- rejoice in it!

Even when we've learned to self-encourage, our wells of self-encouragement can run dry. For me, the best encouragement comes from the LORD. When I cry out to Him- He reminds me that He sees, and gives me peace, safety, comfort, and encouragement to get through.

Keep a journal, even if you are more of a 'jotter' like me, of things (or people) for which you are thankful, things (or people) you found uplifting, inspirational, beautiful, humorous, encouraging, strengthening; perhaps quotes, maxims, Scripture verses… jot the date next to it.

Strength

As with courage, those of us battling ongoing conditions don't always hear that we are strong; after all, we might not have even gotten out of bed the whole day! But, take it from me -I know- just keeping in the battle takes strength! *Be en-couraged!*

Who, and what, encourages you?

Who do you know that brings strength to you? (Invite them to visit, and - *thank them for bringing that strength to your life~)*

Who are other people you know that inspire you with their courage?

When you are able, write that encouraging person a quick note to let them know how they've inspired or encouraged you~ (jot down here, who, and what date you sent off a note)

Look for quotes, or Scripture verses, that bring you encouragement and strength- write them here so you can go right to them on those days you need to 'self-encourage':

HINT: *Check with your local library to see if they have any digital books, biographies and autobiographies, of others who have persevered through difficulties.*

Make a list here of the audio books you'd like to borrow and listen to:

HINT: *If there are people in your life that 'drain you', even on a healthy day; you have permission to set a boundary and not have them visit until* *you are stronger. You can simply say that you just aren't 'strong enough right now' for the visit. Perhaps a caregiver can act as a 'shield' for you and communicate this boundary for you. It can be done graciously and politely, while still giving you the recovery space you need to get stronger.*

Medicinal Music

If you are not bothered too much by sound, you may want to incorporate listening to music into you recovery days. (If you decide to listen to music while bathing- be sure that you keep any electronic devices away from any water!)

···

Pick out music that is soothing; you may even put on a recording of nature sounds, such as from the ocean, forest, songbirds;

try out some classical music, instrumental music, praise and worship music... Whatever is most uplifting and soothing to you.

Some days, you may want something more upbeat and energizing.

Some days, even the slightest noises are bothersome- use ear plugs if necessary.

On the Internet, you may try out listening to *Pandora*™ for free, personalizing the music choices to those you enjoy. Your local library has a good selection of music on CDs you can borrow too.

···

HINT: *If you know of someone who lives nearby, and frequently goes to the library- you may ask them if they'd be willing to drop-off and pick-up items from the library for you. Many library systems will allow you to* *order your library books online; or you may call your local library and ask them if you can order by phone, or if they have a mobile library that comes to your area.*

What are some of your favorite music genres?

Who are your favorite music performers?

What are some of your favorite music titles?

HINT: *Keep your lists of music, book, magazine preferences updated and handy, so when someone is available to get them for you, you will have a ready list for them; which they will appreciate, as for many- their offer comes just as they are heading out to the library.*

■■■

If you are experiencing sensitivities to sounds/music- it is important to communicate this to your caregivers:

What volume setting is most comfortable for you?

What sounds bother you the most right now?

What audio devices do you prefer to use, and where do you use them most (do you have a remote control for the device nearby)?

De-cluttering

When we are ill, we have little energy for keeping things tidy; but as you are able, attend to de-cluttering your most lived in spaces.

Perhaps it is your bedside, couch-side, chair-side; taking the energy to tidy up these areas, even a little, can make a big difference.

If you can be up to any degree, and married, you might ask your spouse, "If I were to only get one thing cleaned or put away today, what would you like me to do?"

Not only will you feel good about 'accomplishing something', but your effort will be appreciated by your family.

• • •

HINT: *If they request a job that is too big for you, let them know you will do it as you can; or part of it. Say they want the bathroom clean, and that is too big of a job for you…then, if you can, choose one aspect of cleaning the bathroom to do at a time. Or, tell them you aren't up to cleaning the whole bathroom, but what part of the bathroom would they most liked cleaned regularly-like the mirrors, the sink…*

• • •

Depending on how you are feeling, you may want to make a goal of de-cluttering some area, perhaps that day, or over the course of a week or month.

HINT: *Ideas for de-cluttering may be: sort the mail, sort magazines, one drawer, one file in the desk… Sort to: throw out, save, give away, or to come back to…*

• • •

By de-cluttering your recovery space- your recovery space will become more peaceful.

• • •

HINT: *Use space on the next page to jot down doable de-cluttering ideas; once you've done them, put the date of completion next to it. It is encouraging to see the page fill up! No job is too small!*

While feeling very ill, but wanting to de-clutter an area- I asked a friend (who had previously offered help if I ever wanted it) who had similar tastes as my own. I got sorting boxes ready and labeled, and set them around the chair I sat in. (I had to label the boxes before I started, because of my brain fog- I wouldn't remember which box was which!)

My friend would get the items from the shelf for me, and when I couldn't decide which box the item should go into, she would help me think it through- and I would take breaks as I needed. She was glad to help, I was glad to get the project done, and the company was wonderful!

What is the area in which you spend most of your healing time?

What is one thing that you can de-clutter in your healing space?

What one thing to de-clutter/clean, is the most appreciated by your family?

What can you do to keep your healing space de-cluttered? (ie, keep wastebasket nearby, limit myself to only 3 magazines or books to gather at a time, keep notes in a notebook instead of on separate pieces of paper...)

My de-cluttering projects: remember, no job is too small!

Self De-cluttering

Not only can our surroundings get cluttered. So can our inner-lives. Long term illnesses have a way of bringing issues to the surface, even those we were sure that we'd buried away. We can have many challenging thoughts and emotions that pile on to everything else we are going through while trying to recover.

Not to mention, that many us with Lyme Disease have endocrine and CNS issues due to the infections, that really mess with our mental health... and is not well understood by our health care providers, counselors, or caregivers...

I was surprised how many issues rose up during the many months of 'grey-scale days', feeling like I was in a mental and emotional 'notherland', or roller coaster. Sometimes issues would come up through dreams, through thoughts; or I'd find myself acting out emotionally toward my family members without even knowing why...

In part this happens because you may no longer have the emotional stamina to keep the issues locked up; it may also happen because of medications; or because of the effects of the infections on your hormones, brain...; simple fatigue and pain can exacerbate emotional wounds...

On top of all the emotional heaving from the illness, our lives... many of us will deeply experience losses from being so ill that will translate into grieving- bringing another dimension to our emotions.

Grief gets so entangled with all the rest of what is going on- that it may not be recognized as grief- but it is important to recognize it and allow yourself to work through the grief process.

There are different 'models of grief' out there... I prefer the 7-Stage grief model. The stages in this model are: Shock & Denial, Pain & Guilt, Anger & Bargaining, 'Depression'-Reflection-Loneliness, the 'Upward Turn', Re-construction & Working Through, Acceptance & Hope. (These are taken from a website: www.recover-from-grief.com)

Sometimes just recognizing you are grieving is a help; people who are grieving tend to journey through these stages of grief sometimes find it is a 'two-step-forward, one-step-back' process- but the important thing is to continue to move forward in the journey. If you find you are getting 'stuck'- seek wise counsel from someone who can help you through the process.

HINT: *There are some practical tools to help you through grief at the website noted above.*

•••

If you are experiencing mental health challenges- first accept that these emotions and thoughts are happening, and pay attention to them. Not only are you going through a time of physical recovery- but it can also be a time of emotional recovery as well.

•••

Jot down any thoughts and emotions that keep coming to mind, write out, or tell someone, about how you are feeling about these things. Journaling and talking with a trusted friend or counselor can be very helpful.

If you are struggling with spiritual issues, or a wounded spirit- you may want to ask for a visit from your pastor; and some churches have professional counselors on staff.

Let your doctor know about any emotional/mental health issues you are experiencing- you may need an adjustment in medications or supplements.

•••

Another good resource is to inquire about a Stephen's Minister. Stephen's Ministry has trained layperson volunteers, who through a local church, will come alongside of you- to visit you and lend a listening ear. If you desire it, they will pray with you as well. They are not professional counselors, but are good listeners and encouragers. There is no fee for a Stephen's Minister.

...

Many churches have Faith Community Nurses- a FCN can visit with you and help you to find community resources for which you may be in need. There is no fee for visiting with a FCN.

...

Your Health Care Provider's office may also direct you to Mental Health resources in your area.

...

HINT: *Try to think of simple 'pick me ups' that you can do- praying, listening to Scripture, talking with a friend, sending someone else a note of encouragement, putting on a team jersey, watching humorous shows/movies through your library/TV/Computer ....There are more ideas throughout this handbook...*

...

What is one personal care habit that when done, really makes you feel 'human' again? *(washing hair, brushing teeth, bathing, favorite piece of clothing...)*

What TV shows or movies make you laugh?

During an ongoing illness, you may discover 'emotional clutter'. What are emotions, perhaps with memories, that you are dealing with? *(If you find there are any that you need help to move through- seek out a trusted friend, pastor, or counselor; journaling can be a good tool for emotional healing...)*

Is everything with your 'heart' okay? Is there anything in your heart that needs to be dealt with, so you can move toward optimal health?

HINT: *It is easy for us to ruminate over things like- 'will it ALWAYS be like this', 'will I EVER get better', 'will I EVER be able to do ___ again', 'when will I start to feel better'… Keep in the present dear one - that is the best advice I can give you- trust God with the future- do what you need to do today.. Matthew 6:33-34 says "But seek first the kingdom and His righteousness; and all these things shall be added unto you. Therefore, do not be anxious for tomorrow; for tomorrow will care for itself. Each day has enough trouble of its own." (NASB)*

The Lord knows what you need (Matthew 6: 30-32).

■■■

It is normal to be 'emotional' in times like this; especially Lyme-fighters. And, a long-term illness can bring feelings of loss, which can bring you through the emotions of grief.

I was especially affected by all the issues of loss I was going through- I was surprised by the grieving processes I went through; but once I understood I was grieving loss in my life, I was better able then to move through it.

■■■

Again, you are not alone! Many Lyme-fighters deal with these different emotions.

The important thing is to let your Health Care Provider know about these emotions. And again- please talk them through with a family member, trusted friend, pastor, counselor…

You don't have to keep it all inside, you don't have tough-it out, you don't have to go through this alone.

■■■

There are online support groups, on which you can find many others who will know just what you are going through- it is such a relief to finally chat with others who truly understand; and, besides chatting with them, you may also learn valuable tools and tips that can help you through the different things you are experiencing.

•••

This is especially good because it is available to you 24/7 and you don't have to leave home if you have a computer and internet. (www.mdjunt-cion.com is a forum on which you can belong to more than one support group, for many of your health challenges)

•••

You may also search the internet sites to find out if there is a support-group meeting near where you live. It is important to make sure that any support group, in person or online- be one that is healthy, in that the participants are there to offer support, be empathetic and to offer helpful ideas in how to deal with common challenges.

•••

However, if you *EVER* feel overwhelmed with emotions, such as hopelessness, sadness, deep anger, dread, just want everything to 'end or go away', you've had thoughts about ending your life, ending the pain....

•••

If you feel you have no one to turn to, and feel you are being overtaken by suicidal thoughts-

Or, if someone you know needs emotional help, *please call the National Suicide Prevention Lifeline.*

You can reach the Lifeline by dialing:
1-800-273-TALK (8255)

Lifeline service is:
FREE and Confidential - staffed by trained counselors -available 24 hours a day 7 days a week -with support services that can help you.

Note for those TTY Users- use this number: 1-800-799-4TTY (4889)

Lifeline Website: www.suicidepreventionlifeline.org

■■■

List the people, and their contact information, that you know you can count on to help you when you are feeling low:

■■■

Cultivating Thankfulness

It may seem strange to have a section about being thankful, when you feel so ill! But it is one of the most therapeutic techniques of all, and hey- it's cheap!

I'm not talking about 'Polly Anna' thinking here- but rather a sincere thankfulness.

Sometimes it is very difficult to even come up with one thing about which to give thanks- but even one thing is a good start!

It doesn't even have to be for anything really big (although that would be great too). Many times it's the little things that add up to a big thanks anyway.

···

Who do you thank? Start by giving thanks to God- even in these circumstances, you can thank Him for Who He Is, and that He knows what you are going through. He is our Redeemer-Helper; the One Who Will Help us through this journey on this presently sin-laden soil, by giving us a Heavenly perspective.

Also- thank those who care for you, and encourage you; be as specific as you can, especially if something in particular was meaningful… no gesture of goodwill is too small to not warrant a gracious thank you for it. If you are able- communicate your thanks through a short note, an email, a phone call… even a sticky-note will do.

···

HINT: *When you practice thanks-giving, you may be surprised to find that you are the one who is most blessed!*

···

Make lists of thankfulness, put the date, what it is you are thankful for, and to whom you are thankful. It will become a wonderful thing to go back to- on days when you are feeling low, and- days when you are feeling better. They will become marvelous mile-markings to you on this journey.

I started to jot down the names of people who helped me in any way- name, what they did, on which date... Then I would try to get a thank you off to them as soon as I was able, and put a check by that note in my notebook.

This helped me keep track of whom I'd thanked, and it was also a good reminder for me on those days that would come when I felt as if no one really cared.

Often, I feel the pull at my DNA of the "Adam and Eve Principle"(Genesis 3)- my eyes settle only on the things I do not to have, and I become disheartened and dissatisfied;

most importantly, I lose my sight of God's goodness, and the things that I can/do have in my life. I need to keep my eyes open for these blessings- as well as for creatively seeing that there are options in 'my Garden' I'd never seen before~

■■■

You can start your own Thanks-Giving record here:

Things for which I am thankful:

Continuous Prayer

My Higher Power is the Lord Jesus Christ. It is wonderful that I can go to Him in prayer anytime, about anything, for anyone.

Not only does He hear and respond to me, but I can also bring other people and their needs before Him.

I keep a directory of our church-goers nearby and can pray through the directory for those people; I am also on the Prayer Line, receiving prayer requests; I pray for family members…

Not only does praying glorify the Lord and benefit me- but it is wonderful to know that even at my weakest, I can be participating in the powerful act of prayer for others, interceding on their behalf.

There have been plenty of days where all I've had energy to pray is, "JESUS!"

God isn't concerned with having a 'lovely-flowery' prayer. He is concerned that we approach Him authentically, humbly, and with anticipation and expectation of His hearing our prayer and that He will answer.

• • •

Some of His answers come quickly; some we don't see evidence of in our lifetime. But, His promise to us is that He does hear and He does care. I was recently challenged by a preacher who asked, 'How would you live if you lived not only knowing God knows you, and cares about you, but that you *live your life like you know it?*'

• • •

Matthew 6:28-34 is a good passage on this…I'll start at verse 31, "*So don't worry about these things, saying, 'What will we eat? What will we drink? What will we wear?' These things dominate the thoughts of unbe-lievers, but your heavenly Father already knows all your needs. Seek the Kingdom of God above all else, and live righteously, and he will give you everything you need.*

So, don't worry about tomorrow, for tomorrow will bring its own worries. Today's trouble is enough for today."

Can I get an "Amen"?!

• • •

Through my own health challenges- the LORD is teaching me to embrace the present- not to fret over what is done, or what might be, or what may not be... Any future plans I make are now written in pencil usually; on a rare occasion, perhaps in erasable ink.

Part of God's will for me is to be dependent on Him, allowing Him to direct my path...ongoing health challenges give me the opportunity to better live in this will of God perhaps even more than some of my healthy friends. Throughout Psalm 37 you can find many verses which apply, like verses 23-24 *"The LORD directs the steps of the godly. He delights in every detail of their lives. Though they stumble, they will never fall, for the LORD holds them by the hand."*

• • •

It is such a comfort to me to know that I don't have to have it all together to go to God; He wants me to come to Him with everything.

I can come to Him because of Who He Is, not because of who I am or what I've done. (If I am coming to Him because of *what I've done*, it is usually to ask His *forgiveness*.)

Many people, especially those who are ill, question what God's will is. Scripture tells us:

"Always be joyful. Never stop praying. Be thankful in all circumstances, for this is God's will for you who belong to Christ Jesus." 1 *Thessalonians 5:16-18 NLT*

This may sound strange and new to you, but being joyful is not dependent on our emotions, or our circumstance. Happiness is something we feel that is mostly dependent on our circumstances.

Joy comes through the unchanging knowledge of the Person of Jesus Christ. *He is* joy, strength, courage, kindness, security, knowledge, peace… We can only truly know these things through Him, not in and of ourselves.

It isn't about our circumstances- even healthy people have incredible challenges to face… It is about living in community with God, getting to know Him more and more, no matter what we are going through.

We can practice joy even when feeling unwell. This is *not* to say that when you are feeling angry, or in pain… that you have to cover that up- but rather acknowledge it, and tell God about it... let Him work in your life.

Joy comes from knowing God, and being in His presence.

"…the joy of the Lord is your strength." *Nehemiah 8:10 NLT*

My hope for you is that you will come to know this Truth personally, not only while in your illness, but unto your wholeness.

•••

Let me take this opportunity to share with you how to begin a personal relationship with Jesus Christ. First, admit you are a sinner by nature and need His forgiveness, recognize that His death on the cross was payment for your personal sin-debt, ask Him to forgive you of your sin nature, and allow Him to internally cleanse you with His forgiveness by inviting Him to do it...Thank Him~

Commit your life to learning about His ways and following His ways by reading the Bible, regularly attending a church that teaches the Gospel and from the Bible, get into a Sunday School group or 'small group' of Christians who get together to learn about God, and to fellowship (hand out in community) with each other. (While healing- you may find Fellowship on the internet through sermons and discussions; or by having a pastor visit...)

Romans 5:7-9 "For one will hardly die for a righteous man; though perhaps for the good man someone would dare even to die. But God demonstrates His own love toward us, in that while we were yet sinners, Christ died for us. Much more then, having now been justified by His blood, we shall be saved from the wrath of God through Him."

1 Peter 3:18 in the Bible says: "Christ died for sins once for all to bring you to God."

John 1:12 says: "To all who received Him, to those who believed in His name, He gave the right to become children of God."

Revelation 3:20 "Jesus said, "Here I am! I stand at the door and knock. If anyone hears My voice and opens the door, I will come in and eat with him, and he with Me."

1John 5:11-12 "God has given us eternal life, and this life is in His son. He who has the Son has life; he who does not have the Son of God does not have life."

A sample prayer is: "Lord Jesus, please forgive my sins, be my Saviour and Lord, unto the gift of eternal life." Amen.

If you prayed this prayer today- note this by recording the date/place _____ And now share this Good News with someone~ (I'd love to hear from you!)

My things to pray about, people to pray for: (thank and praise Him for who He is, my needs, my concerns, prayer for others)

Care-giving Tips
Suggestions to help you care for yourself, or for a loved one.

Juggling all the protocols for someone who is seriously ill can be a challenge for anyone- but especially so for those of us who already have brain fog, and are weak.

···

There is no perfect system for keeping track of medications, supplements, dietary needs, Rife machine treatments, activities, symptoms, doctors, pharmacies… *but a working system must be developed.* You will save yourself a lot of stress in doing so.

The following will give ideas of things you may want to include in a Personal Care Record. The best way to put together and use a Personal Care Record, is by doing it however it works best *for you to use!*

A filing system, a notebook, folders, calendar (day, week, month..), making check off lists, graphing… Be creative. There isn't a 'right or wrong' in *how* you do it, the important thing is: *you do it!*

Developing a Personal Care Record

To keep track of daily meds, supplements, dietary schedule… develop a Personal Care Record with areas for:

Morning

Breakfast

Mid-morning

Lunch

Mid-afternoon

Dinner

Mid-evening

Bedtime

Goals

Notes/Other *(doctor appointments, visitors)*

Fill in any routine items, then, make copies of that sheet. You may choose to use these sheets daily, weekly, monthly...

•••

At the beginning of treatments, it may be most helpful to plan on using it daily. Update as needed. As you improve, you may go to weekly, or monthly Personal Care Records.

•••

Date the sheets for when you use them. In the 'Notes' area- fill-in any comments about:

Effects of treatments

Any symptoms needing note (including intensity using 1-10 scale)

Activities, any changes to routine

Detoxifying bath rotation

Any questions you have (to ask your doctor at next visit)

Note if getting low on any supplements or meds (then note on calendar when you need to re-order)

Note temperature (particularly morning, afternoon, late evening- especially if endocrine system involvement is an issue; or if you have had a history of fevers)

If using a Rife machine- note date, frequencies used, length of time for each frequency, note any reactions-and when you have them

HINT: *You can make up your own Personal Care Records- put it on computer (note in Resource Section on page 137, you can find links to downloadable charts); begin putting the information in a 3-ring binder, or portable file, and keep all your records together.*

•••

By keeping records, it will not only help you to keep everything straight (like what to take when, because this has to be taken before eating, or this one two-hours after eating, or not with probiotics, or minerals…)

Note who you spoke to, about what and when.

It will also be a great tool for your caregivers, and to bring with you to your next doctor's appointment. It can give your health care practitioner valuable information that will better help to formulate your care plan.

•••

It will also be a good 'reality check' for you on those days when you wonder if anything is getting better- you may well note that last month such-n-such was bothering you a lot, according to your notes, but *lo-and-behold*, you haven't had that issue now for weeks!

Over time, the Personal Care Record can give you a good idea of any patterns or trends you are experiencing.

•••

I can remember at the beginning, just getting in my supplements, meds and treatments was an overwhelming prospect, and it took all of my mental and physical energy!

Being I had no small children at home, I had to lay out my meds and supplements on the counter, on a long sheet of paper which had my schedule of meds and supplements...

I would literally have to 'move the bottle' along the schedule list once I had taken it; because, being so forgetful- I could take the med, turn away- and not remember if I had taken it!

•••

HINT: *GET A KITCHEN TIMER!* My kitchen timer has been a life saver to help me remember things like:

- *when* to take a medication
- *when* it had been long enough since taking a med so that I could eat
- *and* to remind me of something-anything else I was supposed to do!
- I could also set my cell phone alarm for a few of the routine medications.

• • •

HINT: *Make sure you do talk to your health care practitioner, pharmacist, supplement manufacturer, homeopathic provider.... about all the different treatments and protocols you are doing.*

You will want to make sure that you are implementing them in such a way that they are working in concert with each other, and to avoid situations where you may be nullifying or even complicating them!

• • •

If you haven't already- make sure that you have a current Health Care Directive filled out. It is important for you to communicate your values and wishes with your family and caregivers.

Keep copies of your Health Care Directive where family members can find it easily; also, see to it that each of your Health Care Providers has a copy.

If at any time, your wishes change- make sure to let your loved ones know, make out a new Directive, and make sure your Health Care Providers replace the old one with the new Directive.

• • •

Also- keep an informal notebook page of care information that you would want your caregiver, in any situation, to know about you. *(Like, I have difficulty swallowing- I would like my caregiver to know that, and should I be hospitalized, I'd like my caregiver to communicate that with the hospital staff.)*

This can relieve your mind to know that even when you may not have the energy to express your needs/desires- you already have a tool in which you have expressed things that are important to you for them to know.

And it is a helpful tool for loved ones who want to help you! If you do not have the strength to fill it out now- ask for help in doing it.

You can start by using this handbook to fill in the information (or ask someone to fill it in as you give the information). Later, you can copy the information into a notebook, or computer…making sure your caregivers each have a copy, or know where the information is.

●●●

Things you may include in your notes are, your:

Full name

Birth date

Insurance information

Health Care Providers (all of them, and what aspect of your care they are a part of, ie- LLMD, NP, PT..)

Primary Physician

The Clinic/Hospital with whom you are associated

Important/often called names & phone numbers *(you may note here any volunteers and what they have offered to help you with; like- Sally, bring a meal. Sandy- cleaning. Judith- ride to doctor.)*

Allergies

Food Intolerances or allergies

Dietary needs (likes, dislikes, not-supposed-to-haves, trouble swallowing)

Beverages that help you detoxify

Pain relieving preference

Type of bath that helps you most for detoxifying

Treatments

Exercises

What kind of massage do you most enjoy- foot, body, shoulders, back etc.

What helps you most if chilled?

What helps you most if running a fever?

Mobility issues- *(dizzy when you get up, need help to tub, certain shoes, help walking, need a cane…)*

How many pillows do you need to re-position, where do you want them placed…

Any position that is intolerable for you *(lying down, a certain side..)*

What things do you like to have near you (*tissues, wastebasket, water/ glass, timer, magazine, TV remote, radio, MP3 player, telephone, pen/ pencil, book, Bible...*)

What is your favorite blanket/pillow...

Do you prefer the room darkened, or drapes open...

What kind of light do you prefer-

Do you want music/TV on/off (*If on, what kind of music, or TV shows*)

Are you allergic to cut flowers? (What are you favorite flowers/colors/ plants…)

Current visitors list- *(if there are people you are not up to seeing while you are recovering, it is ok to ask your caregiver to shield you from them for this time)*

Preference for visitors, update as you need- (*Do you want visitors, prefer phone calls, or letters, emails…What time of day is best for you to receive visitors…*)

Personal Health History

Family Health History

Any other 'comforts' or 'concerns' that you would want someone to know:

HINT: *Be sure to update this information when there are any changes or additions.*

Choosing Healthcare Practitioners & Healthcare Options- **things to consider**

Choosing your Health Care Practitioner isn't always easy; and when you are very ill, it can be even more difficult and confusing. To help with this process, it can be helpful to think through some things, which I will go into here.

By coming to your conclusions about these matters, you will find that wading through the waters of the sea of health care options can be navigated more easily; having these things in mind will help direct you to the care you most desire.

•••

Values - Your values are a stabilizing force in choosing health care options, and yet not often addressed consciously. All of us hold to certain values which direct us through life- and they are an important part of our choosing health care options as well; whether it be choosing a Practitioner or treatments…

···

… identifying your personal and medical values is important. Here are some questions to consider. I invite you think about these and jot down your answers here:

How do my values/spiritual/religious views and convictions impact choosing my health care options? (list out specific spiritual values/ convictions, and those medical practices that they would impact)

What are medical practices that you know of that you would believe to be in conflict with your spiritual values/convictions?

What are medical practices that you believe align with your spiritual values/convictions?

What are the non-negotiable values that would be important to you for your Health Care Practitioner to hold as well (even if you don't hold same religious convictions)?

What are your values when it comes to different Health Care Options?

(There are many options these days- emphasizing different aspects of Health Care- chiropractic, nutriceuticals, homeopathy, Western Medicine, Eastern Medicine, kinesiology, acupuncture, Rife.... Make a list of which you are comfortable with, would be willing to try, need to investigate, absolutely not an option...)

What are other Health Care values that are important to you?

What is your personal philosophy/conviction regarding healing?

Preferences – Preferences are more changeable than our values, but they still have an impact on giving direction as to our Health Care options. Think of it in terms of 'qualities' you prefer… (maybe character of the person you deal with, or an organization, aspects of either/both…maybe location, aesthetics, how they do or do not relate to your Health Coverage…)

What preferences do you have (and why) in a:

Health Care Practitioner-

Health Care Provider-

Clinic-

Laboratory-

Hospital-

Treatment Center-

Therapy center (physical, occupational…)

Other-

Risk/Benefit Analysis-

Today we can be blessed with many options of treatments; but it can also be confusing- in any area of Health Care we choose. Identifying you Values and Preferences can be a good place to start.

•••

However, there are times when we are looking at intense treatments that we may want, or need, to take another look at our options. A helpful tool may be to apply a Risk/Benefit analysis (sometimes called CBA- Cost-Benefit Analysis).

Many people in the Business World are familiar with the terms Risk/Benefit Analysis; if you are not- here is a simplified explanation: As the title suggests- it is simply noting the known risks/costs of that option, and weighing out against the benefits.

In both of these lists, you may include notations on that which is known, and unknown for consideration.

•••

Once you have gathered as much information as you can (from your Practitioners, online, friends, books... You may begin to process the information.

•••

It can be helpful to write out your information as you begin to weigh it all out. On following pages is a tool to help you with the process.

•••

There may be times when you are too ill, and it is all happening so fast- in these cases, ask for help from a trusted caregiver; one who understands your values and preferences the best, who is willing to dig in to the information for you, and then go over it all with you (or give you a summation).

···

Once you have written out as much of the information and its impacts that you can think of- ask a loved one/caregiver to make their own list, then- compare your lists.

(This helps 'widen' your view, and open communication between you and your caregiver as to your approach in choosing treatment options.)

···

Remember, along the way, you may learn new information- you can make the adjustments on your analysis sheet, and determine if the new information is impactful enough to weigh more heavily one way or another and affect your outcome decision.

···

When possible, you may seek out others who have gone through similar treatments to get their input (although everyone reacts differently).

···

HINT: *I have found that the online support group site can be helpful for this. But, I don't take just one or two opinions/experiences.*

I scan through the responses- looking for any patterns of repetition in the responses; i.e., I am looking to see consistently good responses to particular treatments, or responses that are negative or non-existent.

Doing this can give me a wider view. If I see a treatment has many people specifically raving about its affects- I check it out. Especially if I am seeing those marked responses on more than one site.

There have been times too that I am in the midst of a treatment and have found affirmation of my choice by seeing others have good responses, and hearing what kinds of things they experienced along the way has helped me to stick with it, as I would be experiencing the same things and wondering about it.

●●●

You can also get a sense of what may be coming up for a next level of treatment in reading about others' experiences- and it can give you more time to consider your options before you are confronted with making a treatment decision at your upcoming appointment.

●●●

Here is a sample of what a simple personal Risk/Cost Benefit Analysis tool might look like for you-

Risk/Cost	Benefit	Questions (need more information)
Spiritual Impact		
Emotional Impact		
Physical Impact		

Risk/Cost	Benefit	Questions (need more information)
Mental Impact		
Financial Impact		
Impact on Family (relationships)		
Social Impact (relationships)		
Health Care Coverage Impact		

Risk/Cost	Benefit	Questions (need more information)
Environmental Impact		
Others-		

HINT: *Prayer, for wisdom and guidance... is the best tool you have in navigating your way through all this~*

Goals are Important to Your Recovery

Even if your goal is to take your medicine today- that's great! As you feel better, and have attained that goal, incorporate a new goal... When making your goal, here are things to keep in mind, remember- it is most effective when you are as specific as possible.

Good questions to ask are:

What is it you want to accomplish?

What are steps/resources you need to accomplish it?

What are possible obstacles; how will you overcome those?

When will you do it? *(Have a target time to start, set times to meet your goal, and a time to accomplish/re-evaluate it by)*

How often will you do it? *(Times a day, every day, every week, once a month- be specific)*

Are you reasonably sure it can be accomplished? *(Use a scale of 0% to 100% sure, or rate 1-5 stars- however- be mostly sure you can accomplish it before you begin)*

HINT: *Search online for 'goal setting' or 'action plans'- many sites have free examples & downloads of ideas and templates to find one that works best for you.*

Once you have established the answers to those questions- then record your goals in your Personal Care Record- using the questions above as a guide.

Keep your goals worded as simply as possible once you've got a plan.

It may be a one-time goal, such as:

I will order my medications from the pharmacy.

I will call the pharmacy this afternoon.

I only need to do this once for this med.

I am 95% sure I can do this.

...

Maybe it is a goal to drink more water every day. That may look something like this:

- *I will drink at least 8 glasses (8oz) of water every day.*
- *I will write it on my medication reminder sheet to drink an 8 oz. glass of water when I rise, mid-morning, at lunch, mid-afternoon, suppertime, mid-evening, and when taking the two medication that I am to drink with a full glass of water.*
- *I will keep a special glass (in my case- a bright, fun one), out by my schedule to help remind me as well.*
- *By having it a part of my schedule, I feel 80% sure that I can accomplish my goal.*

...

HINT: *Another note regarding visiting with your Health Care Provider- Before your visit: Gather all your notes and records- note any trends or patterns, new symptoms, changes in symptoms.*

Summarize your notes on a page to bring/give to your doctor. If you bring originals, ask them to make their own copy for your doctor.

...

HINT: *You may want to make a list of symptoms- then daily, weekly, or monthly- place a rating scale (0-10; 0 being no symptom, 10 being hospitalized it's so bad); place date next to entries/updates.*

This will help you see any patterns. This is especially good for those of us whose memories are poor, and changes can be subtle.

●●●

Don't forget to attend to your eye, dental, and chiropractic health as well… Keep these practitioners up to date on any new treatments.

List all the questions you want to ask the doctor together on one page to bring with you. (Give your Health Care Practitioner a copy on which to write his answers for you! Make sure you get your copy back.)

●●●

HINT: *If you are like me, you think of the best questions AFTER you leave the doctor's office! Write them down.*

If they are ones that you need answered right away- call the Health Care Provider's office and ask for the nurse; tell the nurse what your questions are, and if she can get back to you with the answers.

Many practitioners are utilizing emails now for these communications. If the questions/comments are not urgent, and can wait until your next visit, write them in your Personal Care Record Notebook for your next visit.

●●●

Ask your family/friends/caregivers if they've noticed any changes (for better or worse); this can be things like your- mood, energy, sleeping patterns, coloration (*My husband responded to me one time, "Tell him you've looked green!"- which I would not have known, and my doctor appreciated the input!*)...

HINT: *Bring extra sheets of plain paper with you- or your Personal Care Record Notebook. If you doctor uses language you do not understand- ask him to explain it. You can also ask him to write it down for you- or even draw it out for you on paper you can keep.*

My Goals: (include who, what, where, when, how)

Keeping Your Balance

Already, there are several things mentioned in these pages that can help you keep balance through your health journey. But, I would like to give special mention to some things I find a challenge for myself, and others, with long-term health issues.

•••

It can be especially gratifying to finally get a diagnosis, especially if you have been ill for a number of years, as many of us have, before finally putting a name to what's been going on.

It is important to embrace the diagnosis and to begin doing all we can to achieve our optimal health; but too often we go a step further, moving from embracing the diagnosis, to allowing it to becoming our identity - we take 'ownership' of it. We begin to frame our diagnosis with "My..."

Don't get me wrong, it is easy to do, and for some it is just an expression, but insidiously it can become a deeply held claim.

Yes, there are many times our health challenges dominate our life, and at the least it calls us to measure out our day in multiple ways (med schedules, doctor appointments, fatigue…).

•••

But, this doesn't mean that the diagnosis, or what we have to do because of it, has to define who we are. *For years, I would explain to people: 'I manage it, so it doesn't manage me'.*

How this plays out for each of us is very individual. But here are some questions you may ask yourself from time to time, to check your own balance in this area:

In whom, or what, do you place your identity?

How often do you use the word 'my' when telling someone what your diagnosis is, or when telling them about a symptom, or point of discomfort?

To whom do you most often use the term 'my _____'?

Are you managing this health challenge, or is it managing you?

If it is managing you, what can you do to change that around? (mentally, physically, socially, emotionally, spiritually...)

Do you give yourself breaks away from the health challenge in any way? (healthy distractions)

Why might it be important to you to be known by this health challenge?

How can you deal with this health challenge, without letting it become the centerpiece of your life?

What differentiates you as a person? (values, preferences...)

What are things you *can* do, you *can* eat?

One Step at a Time

Just want to mention a few things about diet and exercise. (See resources in the back of the book)

Most of us have many food allergies and intolerances- limiting our food options. For many of us, we have had to make some drastic changes in how we eat.

There are many good resources out there, I will not go into this subject in depth; but I would like to point out considerations for you to pursue.

The most important aspects of dietary needs I've found are **eating things that**:

Do not cause inflammation

Are alkalizing, are low-glycemic

Do not contain mercury

Conservative on certain minerals (like copper...check with your Lyme-literate doctor)

Good source of protein (whey concentrated form, good choice)

Balance intestinal flora with probiotics

*And- **stay away from:** alcohol, sugar, tobacco use...*

Other:

Have your saliva checked for enzymes (you may need to supplement)

...

With a Health Care Practitioner's guidance, determine whether or not you have adequate stomach acid- or if you need to supplement it with ACV, or other formula.

...

Make it enjoyable! Be creative! If you have a creative friend that is good with food- give that person a list of what you can and can-not eat (or give them some ingredients you can eat) and ask them to come up with some enjoyable recipes for you. Write down the reci-pes, and keep them in a recipe file. *(who just popped into your mind? _____when will you call them to talk about this? _____)*

...

Eat with others- even if you have to eat your 'own food'- the social inter-action is important.

Keep meals in single serving sized containers in the freezer when pos-sible- so you can pull out any time you need it.

KISS- Keep It Simple Silly

Juice your vegetables and fruits (you can make frozen treats as well)

Set the table- (helps it feel more like a *real* meal)

HINT: *I have found out that keeping food items simple isn't just energy saving for me- but when only using a few food items and simple seasonings* *(like salt, or lemon juice) I can enjoy a very satisfying meal; or, I may jazz up a meal by trying new seasonings on my 'same old' protein dish or rice (added bonus is that many seasoning have medicinal benefits as well at aesthetic ones!)*

...

As to exercise, be sure to ask your Health Care Practicianer for guidelines before beginning any new activities or exercises. (You may have to ask for specifics if the answer is vague.)

Talk to your Practitioner about a Physical Therapy referral.

A basic guideline may be to be active as tolerated. Don't overdo. Some of us understand this, and some of us don't. If you need something more specific, you need to qualify these guidelines- ask for more specifics- or give the Practitioner examples of an activity you have in mind…

Mainly- if you feel you are *starting* to tire, a symptom is becoming noticeable; your muscles are feeling 'tight', your mind is getting more fuzzy… things like these are signals that it is time to stop and rest.

This can be really tough for a lot of us- we want so much to do something, get something done! And as soon as we have a little window of energy- we want to squeeze as much out of it as we can! Sometimes it is 'worth it'- but usually we overdo even over the more mundane, and it is wiser just to leave it be and rest.

A lot of the time I won't even pick up on the fact that I'm going 'downhill' because I am so focused on the task. At that point, one of my biggest 'tells' comes through getting weepy. That's a sure sign I need to go lie down!

Another 'tell' for me, is my son- he is incredibly good at reading me when I have begun to do too much! It is humbling to have my teenage son, albeit gently, tell me I need to go lie down; but he has always been right in his assessment, and I have learned to take his direction with as much grace as I can- thankful for his caring.

···

Even on days that are spent mostly in a horizontal position- purposefully try moving around a bit...even if it is opening and closing a fist, pointing your toes/feet to ceiling and then forward (good for lymph system), or raising your forearm up and down...

···

For a time, I was using a Rife machine that required me to be by the machine for hours a day. We had it in an extra room which was quiet and had a bunk bed. Stronger days would allow me to sit up in a chair during the treatments- other days found me laid out on the bottom bunk!

Sometimes- just for a change of position, I would lie there and put my legs/ feet into the air, with my feet pushing up against the bottom of the top bunk. It looked silly I'm sure but it felt good too!

Funny thing was that months later I was reading about a yoga pose that is good for lymph drainage- yep, you guessed it! Only they have you scooting up to a wall and putting your legs/feet up against the wall as you lie on the floor for five minutes!

So, if you are able, and don't have a bunk bed- you may want to give it a try. At the least you will get an 'ab' work-out from laughing!

···

If you are able- you may want to put on some music and gently (or as vigorously as you are able) march in place! Maybe you'd enjoy being a conductor or drummer to the music- you can do that while marching, or sitting in a chair. It is great for your upper-body (and more fun than *exercising*).

...

As I have been gaining strength- I dug out some old VHS exercise programs to use. They are very low impact and take little room to do them. On strong days- I do it more vigorously; on days I'm not feeling very strong, I'll just do what I can and adjust my level of intensity to how I am feeling.

I know the infectious organisms attacking my body do not like me to exercise! (All the more reason to exercise! I have to think of it as just another treatment I have to do!)

It brings more oxygen to my systems, helps lessen depression (promotes endorphin release), lifts mood, increases metabolism, balances hormones, sharpens mental abilities, can raise your body temperature...

this motivates me to keep moving to whatever degree I can, and to make it a part of my health care routine just as I would with other treatments!

HINT: The important thing isn't HOW MUCH exercise is done, but most importantly that exercise IS DONE! *(passive exercise is even helpful! Aerobic exercise is not for us at this time...)*

What are activities that you can regularly do?

What can you incorporate into your day to add one more step of activity into your routine?

What questions can you ask at your next doctor's appointment about activities and exercises you can do?

What activities do you best tolerate?

What activities do you most wish to work toward being able to do?

HINT: *Keep a log of your activities! It will be encouraging to see what you are able to do, and see your progression over time. Even if it's 'just' walking across the living room, you are getting in exercise and helping to chase away those infectious organisms!*

Finances

Ugh, if you are like me- this is not a favorite subject. Many of us with health issues have to deal a lot with financial issues, complicated (maybe even drained) because of Health Care costs.

At one time I had great insurance. But, because of an illness, I was directed by my doctor to move back with my parents (I was in my late twenties), as I couldn't care for myself. So I did. It meant moving back to my home state.

Back then, I didn't know that my insurance company would not move with me- so I lost it, and all the great coverage! And you know the rest of the story for those with pre-existing conditions and trying to find insurance (especially 'affordable' insurance)!

Communication is a key component when dealing with finances- this includes: keeping good records; communicating with your Health Care Providers and Practitioners- and their billing departments. Know your insurance company and how to file any claims, what are co-pays, deductibles...

If married- keep open communication with your spouse about any upcoming or incoming medical expenses, in advance if at all possible, try to ball-park monthly expenses for medical needs and budget that amount...

Pay bills as you can, and what you can- just make sure that if you are unable to pay the full amount, let the bill department know of your situation, and how much you believe you can pay at this time/per month.

Seek financial counseling- may be through your church, an accountant, banker, social worker, or an reputable company that gives financial counseling (see resources).

In some areas- there are programs for Lyme patients who may qualify for discounts on medications. Check with your local Lyme Support Group, or online.

Buy generic whenever possible. Shop online to see if there are better deals. Consolidate supplement orders by phone, or online, to save shipping costs. It sometime pays, and makes life easier to have some supplements or meds sent automatically.

Check with a local tax preparer to find out what records to keep, regarding your medical expenses, which may be deductible on next year's taxes. (Like mileage to, and from, doctor appointments...)

Mileage log:

My Story (part B)
a few things I am learning along the way...

While I was in the throes of illness and treatments, my family took on roles of caregivers. Each one, though not consciously, approached their care-giving role uniquely.

One person wasn't doing it all (although my husband carried the greatest weight), but each one's approach to helping suited who they are, and met my needs in different ways.

Early on, I would get frustrated that none of them could 'read my mind' as to what I needed when I was most ill.

Later, I realized that none of them had health care backgrounds, and it was silly of me to think they would see those kinds of things that needed to be done. Even if they *did have* a health care background- I needed to do a better job communicating my needs to them!

As I could- I made up my own Care Plan to which any of them could refer if they needed, or wanted to. I felt better just knowing that I had a tool to communicate what my needs were on a daily basis.

I also had to realize that everyone deals differently with people who are ill. My husband had to point this out to me.

I knew this was true- but I had assumed because I was a nurse by nature, and because we were family, that family would intuitively know how to care for me, and know what I needed.

I was wrong! And by being wrong in my assumptions- I caused a lot of angst to myself and my family.

I would encourage you:

    a. Don't assume someone, even a loved one, knows what you need

    b. Communicate your needs

    c. Allow the other person to be who they are. (If they are unable to give you care, love them anyway; think of, and ask for, someone else you know who can help you).

•••

Not all family members are built to be caregivers- no matter how much you, or they, want them to be. If that is the case, as I said, love them anyway. Then on your own, or with a loved one, or the help of someone else (through the church, support resource) find someone who is available to help you.

 Keep in mind, your family is usually doing so much more at this point anyway, trying to keep things going, that they are also stressed and pulled in many directions with the additional load.

•••

Don't expect one person to be able to provide for all your needs. The more you accept help from others, the more you will find that each individual brings another aspect of caring to your world.

•••

When we are ill, our world 'shrinks'- and it is easy to lose perspective. Don't forget to thank those who help you. Balance out asking for help, and doing for yourself as you are able to do so.

Try to consolidate your requests as much as possible- keep a pad and pencil close by to make a list of things you think of for when your helper comes.

Find ways to encourage your caregivers- ask them about their life; ask them how you can be praying for them (jot their prayer requests down so you don't forget them; ask them later for an update).

Ask your caregiver what times work best for them- then work your treatment schedules, or whatever is negotiable or nonessential, around them as much as possible.

...

Say you had terrible night sweats again, your bed was soaked. You'd like fresh linens put on that morning. But, your caregiver's best time to do it isn't until later that day... then graciously tell them thank-you and that you are looking forward to it.

My husband has had to make plenty of trips to the grocery for me- and it isn't his favorite place to shop. I usually have a list written of items per each isle at our store.

I write my list in my own 'language' for what I will get. (Like 'bread' will mean something to me: whole grain; and to my son it means processed-white *bread!)*

I can easily get upset with my husband about that one item that he got differently than what I wanted- or I can concentrate on his willingness to go to the store for me.

If I am sending someone on an errand for me, and the items is important- I must make sure to adequately describe the item and its importance, other- wise- I must be willing to overlook the item and love the person if it is not just what I wanted.

...

This whole process has been, and is, a time of deepening my relationship with the LORD. Before this current health challenge, I had begun to see how important it was not to concentrate as much on what I needed, or wanted, to change in my life; rather, by concentrating on learning *to know God more deeply*, those things began to change.

Fear for instance. A couple years ago I was impressed with how many of us are leading 'fear-driven lives', instead of 'eternity-driven lives'. If I wanted to deal with my fear- I would have come to God with my fear and asked Him to take it away, or I would've tried behavioral techniques to try to change.

Again, what I have found to be of the most profound and most healing, is to learn more about *who* the LORD is, draw closer to Him. In the case of me being filled with fear, through studying Scripture, I'm learning that He is Trustworthy, Loving, Kind, Gentle, a Strong Tower, Strength, Unchanging, Safety…

And as I meditate on those aspects of who He is, my fear fades, and I experience the security of being in His presence.

This can be applied to when one is lonely, in pain, feeling rejected, feel- ing misunderstood… The Scripture is fraught with passages which tell us who God is, in answer to every emotion and thought of man.

In many Bibles, there is a concordance, usually located in the back of it. There, you may look for a word describing how you feel, and it will direct you to verses in which that word appears. Online, you can also go to www.Biblegateway.com , there you can look up references using a keyword.

You may want to try something I have begun to do, particularly in the book of Psalms. I will read through a Psalm with the purpose of answering the question "What does this passage say about *who* God is?"

As I come upon word describing who He is, I jot that word down in the margin of the text, or in a note book.   I also like to note the date and circumstance of any of those descriptions that hold particular meaning for me, and why.

•••

There is a wonderful full version of C.H. Spurgeon's classic commentary called *Treasury of David*. If you would enjoy a rich study of the book of Psalms, I encourage you to take a look at it. http://www.spurgeon.org/treasury/treasury.htm

•••

I am not a journaler - I call myself a 'jotter'. So, when I am reading Scripture, I just make quick notes- in the margins, or in a little notebook. Others I know fill page after page in their journals. Some are now journaling by recording their thoughts and insights on webcams.

•••

A fellow FCN (Faith Community Nurse), and facebook ™ friend, has been reading through a journal her mother had written in through the years. Mostly it is a journal of her prayer life. They are beautiful, authentic and heartfelt prayers- so many of us can relate to the wise woman's words.

Not only are they a blessing now to her daughter, but to others with whom her daughter now shares them. It is a wonderful gift to us all.

...

If at all possible- make a record of what *you* are learning, and observing in your times of meditation and prayer. It somehow makes what you are learning even more real, and at the very least- it will be a great tool for your own encouragement, as you see God's answers…and who knows, perhaps one day these life-notes may be a part of your own legacy to encourage the generations to come!

...

As I am going through these pages editing, I am now in my 10th month of treatments. There have definitely been improvements- my eye sight is better, I don't have the 'fibro-like' pains, the quality of my muscles has improved, I have less brain fog, the air hunger is gone,

I haven't had night sweats in months, the neck pain is much less (still have soreness from neck injury incurred in the car accident), headaches lessened, I am finally getting through the days without dread – and without feeling like every time I lay down I may not wake up again, my heart rate is more normal… to name *a few*.

Still, I am continuing my treatment protocols, hitting these buggers from as many directions as possible. My doctor had told me it can take years to really know how much I may recover.

I regularly need to remind myself to stay in the present, and look at the big picture. Those times still come when I get that 'sick' feeling and have to rest… it is hard not to be discouraged, or fearful that the infections are gaining ground…

Although I am slowly continuing to improve, there is still the typical waxing-n-waning in the course of the disease and treatment- I need to remember to think in terms of "am I better than last month", and that helps give me perspective.

I must keep my mind reigned in and focused, and keep doing all my treatments – watching what I eat, getting exercise… I must keep disciplined, no matter how much I want to just stop doing *all* this, *all* the time…

I don't want to go back to the days that the infections were ruling me! And so I press on…. We press on!

…

One of the biggest lessons I've been learning, is even when you are at your weakest, unable to do much of anything, *you are still valuable* to God. For our value is not based on what we can do; but instead, it is based on who God is, and what He has done for us. So rest in that, and let your heart rejoice in knowing that the King of Kings knows you, cares about you, He values you!

…

1 Peter 5:7 *"Give all your worries and cares to God, for he cares about you."*

I have been hesitant to include my treatment regime, but others have encouraged me to share it - so I will. However, I will do so with a caution:

Everyone with Lyme presents differently. We have many similarities and hallmarks- but we may have different organisms, and we certainly are different in how our bodies do/do not respond to the organisms and treatments.

By sharing what I have been doing over the course of this year, I am in NO way communicating that this is THE WAY, or that you should do what I am doing!

It is important to keep in contact with your own Lyme Literate doctor, research on your own, find what you want to try/do- keep communication with your Lyme-literate doctor open and with mutual respect in deciding on your personal care plan.

And remember, healing is a process- and with Lyme Disease, it tends to be a LONG process.

...

I will generally, and in brief, share what I have been doing: Minocycline, Hydroxychloroquine, Armour Thyroid, ABARB, ABART, Rife Machine (started on Pro-Gen running through several different Banks of frequencies- at times for 6-8 hours per day)- now using an EMEM5 several frequencies once every one to two weeks. Thorne Basic Nutrients without copper and Iron™, Vitamin C, Quercitin with C, DHEA, CoQ10, Vitamin D3, Phosphaline 4:1 ™, Immunoviva Core ™, Coconut Oil, S-Acetyl Glutathione…

Juicing (to detoxify- using: carrots, celery, lemon juice, cucumbers; to which I add Young Living ™ oils: Lemon, Ginger, Nutmeg, Oregano, Copaiba, Cardamom, Clove, Grapefruit, Cinnamon; for detox baths I use these Young Living oils- Lemon, Wintergreen, Spearmint, Peppermint, Endoflex… Other Young Living oils I use: Lavender, Thieves, Lemongrass, Believe, Purification, …

...

I have many diet restrictions due to Lyme, as well as my personal intolerances and allergies. Key factors are eating habits that include healthy protein intake (I supplement with Whey protein (isolate)- I like teraswhey ™).

...

I take digestive aids digestive enzymes (Digest-Ez™ from Eniva), as well as Metagest™ (Metagenics ™); for lighter snack- 1tsp of ACV with water; probiotics (either through Eniva or Young Living- order information can be found in Resources section). I avoid sugar, and use Stevia ™ as a sugar substitute. I stay away from processed foods as much as possible. Organic meat, veggies, fruit…as possible. For oils- I primarily use Olive oil, coconut oil, and organic butter.

...

For exercise- I've been slowly working out using Leslie Sansone's 'walking' exercise routine DVDs. I can do them at home, and as tolerated. I am also going to Physical Therapy.

...

There are so many good options out there for things such as supplements- there are a lot more supplements I could take- but given the financial distress Lyme has caused me…my doctor is very judicious about keeping it to the essentials for me, which I appreciate.

...

That is one of the realities that many of us have to deal with- as lovely as it would be to get everything we'd like to get, even for our health… health care is very much more a privilege than a right… We do what we can- and give the rest over to God; for ultimately we are all in His care according to His will. I don't always understand it, but it is truth.

...

The most crucial part of my treatments has been:

depending on God, and trusting Him for the outcome to be according to His will;

the support of my family,

and the wonderful prayer support that I have had through my family, friends, church, and community!

RESOURCES

Rest Ministries: www.restministries.org   Lisa Copen author of: *"Why Can't I Make People Understand?" "Mosaic Moments"* (devotions for the chronically ill) "505 Ways to Encourage a Chronically Ill Friend"

www.butyoudontlooksick.com Living with ongoing health challenges.

"Spoons" illustration can be found at this site; it illustrates what it is like to live with an 'invisible' illness.

Note, I did not go into clay baths, although beneficial to your body, they can wreak havoc with you plumbing/drainage system. For more on clay baths- check out "Homemade Detox Baths" by Annie B. Bond- available at www.Lulu.com or www.Amazon.com

"Homemade Detox Baths" also has a great section on Sea Weed Baths. These baths may be especially helpful to those dealing with issues involving their adrenal and thyroid glands.

Another good supplement is Astaxanthin- not only is it a great antioxidant, and has even been reported to help protect your skin from sunburn. http://www.naturalnews.com/Files/Astaxanthin.pdf

Soul Food

Linda Dillow, ***Calm My Anxious Heart- A Woman's Guide to Finding Contentment***, Colorado Springs, Colorado, NavPress Publishing Group, 1998 ISBN: 1-57683-047-0

Carol Kent, ***Tame Your Fears- and Transform Them into Faith, Confidence, and Action***, Colorado Springs, Colorado, NavPRess Publishing Group, 1993,2003   ISBN: 1-57683-359-3

Erwin W. Lutzer, ***Putting Your Past Behind You- Finding Hope for Life's Deepest Hurts*** *(Revised)*, Chicago, Illinois, Moody Publishers, 1997 ISBN-13: 978-0-8024-5641-1

Charles Stanley, ***The Blessings of Brokenness- Why God Allows Us To Go through Hard Times***, Grand Rapids, Michigan, ZONDERVAN Publishing, 1997 ISBN: 0-310-20026-1

Lisa J. Copen, ***Why Can't I Make People Understand? Discovering the validation those with chronic illness seek and why***, San Diego, California, Rest Ministries Publishers, 2005 ISBN: 978-0-9716600-4-2

Erwin Raphael McManus, ***Uprising- A Revolution of the Soul***, Nashville, Tennessee, Thomas Nelson, Inc., 2003, ISBN: 0-7852-6431-0

Erwin Raphael McManus, ***Chasing Daylight***, Nashville, Tennessee, Thomas Nelson, Inc, 2002, ISBN:0-7852-8113-4

Ann Voskamp, ***one thousand gifts- A DARE TO LIVE FULLY RIGHT WHERE YOU ARE,*** Grand Rapids, Michigan, Zondervan, 2010, ISBN: 978-0-310-32191-0

Andy Stanley, ***Enemies of the Heart- Breaking Free from the Four Emotions that Control You,*** Colorado Springs, Colorado, Multnomah, 2006 & 2011, ISBN: 978-1-60142-145-6

Byron Katie & Hand Wilhelm, *Tiger-Tiger is it True,* Carlsbad, CA, Hay House USA, ISBN: 978-1-4019-2560-4

Devotionals:

Sarah Young, Jesus Calling –Enjoying Peace in His Presence- Devotions for Every Day of the Year, Nashville, Tennessee, Thomas Nelson, Inc, Publisher, 2004 ISBN: 978-1-59145-188-4

www.Biblegateway.com

Max Lucado, *Grace for the Moment, vol II- More Inspirational Thoughts for Each Day of the Year*, Nashville, Tennessee, J Countryman- a Division of Thomas Nelson, Inc, Publisher 2006 ISBN: 1-40410-097-0

Dean F. Ridings, *the Pray! Prayer JOURNAL- Daily Steps Toward Praying God's Heart*, Colorado Springs, Colorado, NavPress Publishing , 2003   ISBN: 978-1-57683-616-3

http://www.spurgeon.org/treasury/treasury.htm Treasury of David, CH Spurgeon

http://breakawayministries.org/resources/podcast   Ben Stuart podcasts

http://northpoint.org/messages   Andy Stanley messages (check: "It Came From Within")

Lisa J. Copen, Mosiac Moments- Devotions for the Chronically Ill – Spiritual Glue for Those feeling Crushed in Spirit, San Diego, California, Rest Ministries Publishers, 2011   ISBN: 978-097-1660038

Lyme Disease

Dr. Nicola McFadzean, *The Lyme Diet- Nutritional Strategies for Healing Lyme Disease*, South Lake Tahoe, California, www.LymeBook.com, 2010 ISBN: 978-0-9825138-3-5

Kenneth Singleton, MD, The *Lyme Disease Solution,* 2008

Bryan Rosner, *When Antibiotics Fail...Lyme Disease and Rife Machines- with Critical Evaluation of Leading Alternative Therapies,* www.LymeBook.com, 2004   ISBN: 0-9763797-0-8

Bryan Rosner, The Top 10 Lyme Disease Treatments, 2007

Karen Vanderhoo-Forschner, Everything You Need to Know About Lyme and Other Tick Borne Diseases, 2003

Burton A. Waisbren, Treatment of Chronic Lyme Disease: 51 Case Reports and Essays, 2011

Stephan Harrod Buhner, Healing Lyme: Natural Healing and Prevention of Lyme Borreliosis and Its Co-Infections, 2005

http://www.lymebook.com/recipes-for-repair-cookbook-piazza   Gail and Laur Piazza, Recipes for Repair Cookbook, 2010

Pamela Weintraub, Cure Unknown: Inside the Lyme Epidemic, 2008

Denise Lang with Kenneth Liegner, MC, Coping with Lyme Disease: A Practical Guide to Dealing with Diagnosis and Treatment, 2004

Of Power and Love and Sound Mind: Six Years with Undiagnosed Lyme Disease, 1989

Many other books about Lyme Disease can be found at www.lymebook. com

Related information

Deitrich Klinghardt, MD, PhD, has many articles and books out about Lyme, as well as Co-Infections and dealing with mold issues.

Dr. Shoemaker has great information on dealing with mold, and crossover with Lyme Disease http://www.survivingmold.com/

Check to see if there is a **"Chronic Disease Self-Management Program"** (Stanford University) being held in your area. You can ask your County Public Health Office, or Clinician's Office.

www.Biblegateway.com

www.pandora.com

Blogs

http://www.susielarson.com/blog/

http://www.aholyexperience.com/

www.encouragementforlymefighters.blogspot.com

Online Support groups:

www.mdjunction.com There is a Lyme Support group, as well as a group for Teens with Lyme

Lyme info websites:

http://info.lymebook.com/profile2.html Herx

http://www.lymediseaseblog.com/jarisch-herxheimer-reaction-lyme-disease/Herx

http://www.ilads.org great Lyme site, lots of info

http://www.environmentalmedicineinfo.com/ health and your personal environment/Multiple Chemical Sensitivity

Mold & marriage- affects on http://www.ei-resource.org/expert-columns/dr.-lisa-nagys-column/household-mold-and-marital-discord/

http://www.faithradionet.com/wp-content/uploads/2011/10/LTP-Monday-10-3-11.mp3   Brandilyn Collins interview/experience with Lyme

Dr Jemsk   speaking on Lyme   http://www.youtube.com/watch?v=V-lHDA863TM&feature=player_embedded#

http://www.lymediseaseblog.com/how-lyme-disease-affects-immune-system/

http://www.lymediseaseblog.com/getting-rid-of-lyme/

http://www.lymediseaseblog.com/lyme-disease-symptoms/

http://www.lymediseaseblog.com/resources/

http://turnthecorner.org/ is now: www.tbdalliance.org

http://www.ilads.org/lyme_disease/lyme_tips.html

http://www.ilads.org/lyme_disease/B_guidelines_12_17_08.pdf

http://www.ilads.org/lyme_research/chronic_lyme.html

http://www.prohealth.com/library/showarticle.cfm?libid=16301

Bio-terrorism/conspiracy theory: http://www.edieclark.com/journey

_into_the_heart_of_lyme_disease_64093.htm

http://www.squidoo.com/history-oflyme-disease

Late Stage Lyme/info/encouragement: http://www.angelfire.com/me2/StarShar/Herx1.html Herx

Mental health assessment for Lyme: http://www.mentalhealthandillness.com/tnaold.html

www.lymedisease.org (Formerly California Lyme Disease Association)

www.lymediseaseassociation.org

http://www.hopeismyanchor.com/Lyme.html   Lots of links listed on this site~

Herbal formulas Byron White- http://www.byronwhiteformulas.com/

Financial help with Rx expenses: http://www.lymedisease.org/news/touchedbylyme/prescription_hope.html

Financial aid when available for testing: www.Lyme-tap.com

Lyme and Co-Infections Chart: http://www.lyme-symptoms.com/LymeCoinfectionChart.html

More on Co-Infections: http://www.lymedisease.org/lyme101/coinfections/ other_tick_diseases.html

MN Lyme Support http://www.mnlyme.com./about_us

Real, even if controversial- story of person with Lyme http://www.washingtonpost.com/national/health-science/the-doctor-diagnosed-chronic-lyme-disease-but-many-experts-say-it-doesntexist/2012/02/06/gIQA4aMHtR_story.html

Resource for first timers being tested for Lyme who have financial challenges: http://www.lymetap.com/

Helpful Informational brochures that can be downloaded/copied/hand out: http://www.ilads.org/lyme_disease/lyme_brochures.html

Lyme Treatment Guidelines http://www.ilads.org/lyme_disease/treatment_guidelines.html

Testing:

80% accurate for Lyme (spirochete):http://advanced-lab.com/spirochete.php

IGENEX- http://igenex.com/Website/

Information regarding NK cells/testing http://www.lymebook.com/lyme-disease-nk-natural-killer-cells

Understanding Western Blot results: http://www.mnlyme.com./yahoo_site_admin1/assets/docs/Understanding_the_lyme_test_results.14291748.pdf

http://www.mdjunction.com/forums/lyme-disease-support-forums/tips/1092391-missouri-drcs-western-blot-explanations-of-nos

Mind Exercises online: http://www.fun4thebrain.com/
and don't forget the games that are already on your computer

Chiropractic care:

NUCCA, Dr. Jeffrey Leach, Living Well Chiropractic , Plymouth, MN
http://www.livingwellmn.com/our-doctors/

Counseling Services:

Focus on the Family- www.focusonthefamily.com 1-800-A-FAMILY

Lutheran Social Services/ Financial Counseling http://www.lssmn. org/ (in Minnesota)

Supplies:

Essential Oils:

www.youngliving.com Quality essential oils. (If you choose to order and need a member number to use, I'd be appreciative if you'd use my number: 868441)

Digestive aids/nutriceuticals: www.enivamembers.com/cynthia #178956

Bath Salts- in bulk http://www.sfsalt.com

Natural lotions/makeup- http://www.ourlemongrassspa.com/2016

Far Infrared Saunas:

www.goodhealthsaunas.com (1-888-99-SAUNA, tell them the Lyme lady at the MN State Fair told you to call)

Caregivers ideas/support:

Lisa J. Copen, *Beyond Casseroles- 505 Ways to Encourage a Chronically Ill Friend*, San Diego, California, Rest Ministries Publishers, 2008 ISBN:0-9716600-6-9

Stephen's Ministries- contact to find Stephen's Ministry in your area, or to learn more about your church developing a Stephan's Ministry: http://www.stephenministries.org/

Faith Community Nurses (Parish Nurses) http://www.efca.org/reach-national/compassion-and-justice/efca-faith-community-nurse-network

http://www.efca.org/reachnational/compassion-and-justice/efca-faith-community-nurse-network

http://www.fcnntc.org/

To learn more about Parish Nurses/Faith Community Nurses: http:// www.queenscare.org/files/qc/pdfs/ParishNursingFactSheet0311.pdf

Charts *(may be downloaded and copied for your own use)*

- Symptoms chart: Pages 9-11 at http://www.ilads.org/lyme_disease/B_guidelines_12_17_08.pdf
- *Medicine distribution chart ideas: http://office.microsoft.com/en-us/ templates/medicine-distribution-chart-and-medical-history-with-emergency-contacts-TC030000162.aspx*
- http://www.heartfailurematters.org/EN/Documents/medicine_chart.pdf
- http://img.webmd.com/dtmcms/live/webmd/consumer_assets/ site_images/media/pdf/hw/form_aa86803.pdf
- http://www.freeprintablemedicalforms.com/category/diaries *Many* Charts available through this site!

Pain management site with downloadable charts: http://www.partnersagainstpain.com/tracking-pain/management.aspx

Record your own favorite/useful resources here:

Contacting the author

If you have something you'd like to share with me about what you have been learning through your own journey, you may contact me via email at: **cdainsberg@ymail.com**

We have much to learn from each other! (However, please keep in mind I will not be able to give you medical advice, or always be able to email you back.)

2 Peter 3:18 "[18] but grow in the grace and knowledge of our Lord and Savior Jesus Christ. To Him *be* the glory, both now and to the day of eternity. Amen."

Ephesians 1:15-21 "[15] For this reason I too, having heard of the faith in the Lord Jesus which *exists* among you and your love for all the saints, [16] do not cease giving thanks for you, while making mention *of you* in my prayers; [17] that the God of our Lord Jesus Christ, the Father of glory, may give to you a spirit of wisdom and of revelation in the knowledge of Him. [18] *I pray that* the eyes of your heart may be enlightened, so that you will know what is the hope of His calling, what are the riches of the glory of His inheritance in the saints, [19] and what is the surpassing greatness of His power toward us who believe.

These are in accordance with the working of the strength of His might[20] which He brought about in Christ, when He raised Him from the dead and seated Him at His right hand in the heavenly *places*, [21] far above all rule and authority and power and dominion, and every name that is named, not only in this age but also in the one to come."

Psalm 71:14 "But as for me, I will hope continually, And will praise You yet more and more."

Psalm 73: 25-26, 28 " Whom have I in heaven but Thee? And besides Thee, I desire nothing on earth. My flesh and my heart may fail, But God is the strength of my heart and my portion forever…. But as for me, the nearness of God is my good; I have made the Lord GOD my refuge, that I may tell of all Thy works."

Benediction

Ephesians 3:14-21 New American Standard Bible (NASB)

[14] For this reason I bow my knees before the Father, [15] from whom every family in heaven and on earth derives its name, [16] that He would grant you, according to the riches of His glory, to be strengthened with power through His Spirit in the inner man, [17] so that Christ may dwell in your hearts through faith; and that you, being rooted and grounded in love, [18] may be able to comprehend with all the saints what is the breadth and length and height and depth, [19] and to know the love of Christ which surpasses knowledge, that you may be filled up to all the fullness of God.

[20] Now to Him who is able to do far more abundantly beyond all that we ask or think, according to the power that works within us, [21] *to Him be* the glory in the church and in Christ Jesus to all generations forever and ever.

Amen.

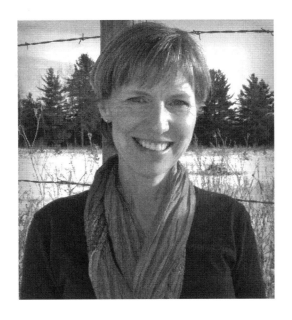

About the Author

Cynthia Dainsberg, RN, FCN (Faith Community Nurse), has lived with chronic conditions for over 25 years- including being a Lyme Fighter since 2011. She is a pastor's wife, mom of three young adults, home educator, and a writer. Cynthia is currently learning to embrace being both an introvert, and a wonk. Some of her hobbies are: keeping it simple, enjoying the beauty of nature, practicing the art of being 'present', baking, and handcrafts. Cynthia lives in a town of 111 people, in a beautiful lake-filled northwoods vacation area.

The Top 10 Lyme Disease Treatments: Defeat Lyme Disease With The Best Of Conventional And Alternative Medicine

By Bryan Rosner
Foreword by James Schaller, M.D.

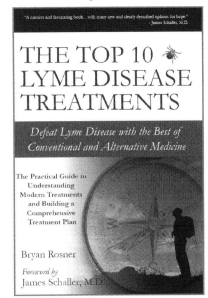

Book • $35

This information-packed book identifies ten promising conventional and alternative Lyme disease treatments and gives practical guidance on integrating them into a comprehensive treatment plan that you and your physician can customize for your individual situation and needs.

The book was not written to replace Bryan Rosner's first book (*Lyme Disease and Rife Machines*, opposing page). It was written to complement that book, offering Lyme sufferers many new foundational and supportive treatment options, based on the author's extensive research and years of personal experience. Topics include*:

- Systemic enzyme therapy, which helps detoxify tissues and blood, reduce inflammation, stimulate the immune system, and kill Lyme disease bacteria.
- Lithium orotate, a powerful yet all-natural mineral (belonging to the same mineral group as sodium and potassium) capable of profound neuroprotective activity.
- Thorough and extensive coverage of a complete Lyme disease detoxification program, including discussion of both liver and skin detoxification pathways. Specific detoxification therapies such as liver cleanses, bowel cleanses, the Shoemaker Neurotoxin Elimination Protocol, sauna therapy, mineral baths, mineral supplementation, milk thistle, and many others. Ideas to reduce and control herx reactions.
- Tips and clinical research from James Schaller, M.D.
- A detailed look at one method for utilizing antibiotics during a rife machine treatment campaign.
- Wide coverage of the Marshall Protocol, including an in-depth discussion of its mechanism of action in relation to Lyme disease pathology. Also, the author's personal experience with the Marshall Protocol over 3 years.
- An explanation of and new information about the Salt / Vitamin C protocol.
- Hot-off-the-press information on mangosteen fruit (not to be confused with mango) and its many benefits, including antibacterial, anti-inflammatory, and anti-cancer properties.
- New guidelines for combining all the therapies discussed in both of Rosner's books into a complete treatment plan. Brief and articulate for consideration by you and your doctor.
- Also includes updates on rife therapy, cutting-edge supplements, political challenges, an exclusive interview with Willy Burgdorfer, Ph.D. (discoverer of Lyme), and much more!

"Bryan Rosner thinks big and this new book offers big solutions."
- James Schaller, M.D.

"Another ground-breaking Lyme Disease book."
- Jeff Mittelman, moderator of the Lyme-and-rife group

"Brilliant and thorough."
- Nenah Sylver, Ph.D.

Do not miss this top Lyme disease resource. Discover new healing tools today! Bring this book to your doctor's appointment to help with forming a treatment plan.

Paperback book, 7 x 10", 367 pages, $35

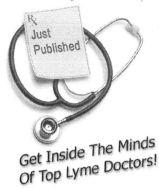

13 Lyme Doctors Share Treatment Strategies!

In this new book, not one, but thirteen Lyme-literate healthcare practitioners describe the tools they use in their practices to heal patients from chronic Lyme disease. Never before available in book format!

**Insights Into Lyme Disease Treatment:
13 Lyme Literate Health Care Practitioners
Share Their Healing Strategies**

**By Connie Strasheim
Foreword by Maureen Mcshane, M.D.**

If you traveled the country for appointments with 13 Lyme-literate health care practitioners, you would discover many cutting-edge therapies used to combat chronic Lyme disease. You would also spend thousands of dollars on hotels, plane tickets, and medical appointment fees—not to mention the time it would take to embark on such a journey.

Even if you had the time and money to travel, would the physicians have enough time to answer all of your questions? Would you even know which questions to ask?

In this long-awaited book, health care journalist and Lyme patient Connie Strasheim

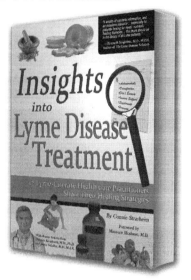

Paperback • 443 Pages • $39.95

has done all the work for you. She conducted intensive interviews with 13 of the world's most competent Lyme disease healers, asking them thoughtful, important questions, and then spent months compiling their information into 13 organized, user-friendly chapters that contain the core principles upon which they base their medical treatment of chronic Lyme disease. The practitioners' backgrounds span a variety of disciplines, including allopathic, naturopathic, complementary, chiropractic, homeopathic, and energy medicine. All aspects of treatment are covered, from anti-microbial remedies and immune system support, to hormonal restoration, detoxification, and dietary/lifestyle choices. **PHYSICIANS INTERVIEWED:**

- Steven Bock, M.D.
- Ginger Savely, DNP
- Ronald Whitmont, M.D.
- Nicola McFadzean, N.D.
- Jeffrey Morrison, M.D.
- Steven J. Harris, M.D.
- Peter J. Muran, M.D., M.B.A.

- Ingo D. E. Woitzel, M.D.
- Susan L. Marra, M.S., N.D.
- W. Lee Cowden, M.D., M.D. (H)
- Deborah Metzger, Ph.D., M.D.
- Marlene Kunold, "Heilpraktiker"
- Elizabeth Hesse-Sheehan, DC, CCN
- Visit our website to read a FREE CHAPTER!

Paperback book, 7 x 10", 443 pages, $39.95

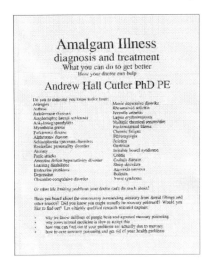

Book • $35

Amalgam Illness, Diagnosis and Treatment: What You Can Do to Get Better, How Your Doctor Can Help

By Andrew Cutler, PhD

This book was written by a chemical engineer who himself got mercury poisoning from his amalgam dental fillings. He found that there was no suitable educational material for either the patient or the physician. Knowing how much people can suffer from this condition, he wrote this book to help them get well. With a PhD in chemistry from Princeton University and extensive study in biochemistry and medicine, Andrew Cutler uses layman's terms to explain how people become mercury poisoned and what to do about it. The author's research shows that mercury poisoning can easily be cured at home with over-the-counter oral chelators – this book explains how.

In the book you will find practical guidance on how to tell if you really have chronic mercury poisoning or some other problem. Proper diagnostic procedures are provided so that sick people can decide what is wrong rather than trying random treatments. If mercury poisoning is your problem, the book tells you how to get the mercury out of your body, and how to feel good while you do that. The treatment section gives step-by-step directions to figure out exactly what mercury is doing to you and how to fix it.

> "Dr. Cutler uses his background in chemistry to explain the safest approach to treat mercury poisoning. I am a physician and am personally using his protocol on myself."
>
> **- Melissa Myers, M.D.**

Sections also explain how the scientific literature shows many people must be getting poisoned by their amalgam fillings, why such a regulatory blunder occurred, and how the debate between "mainstream" and "alternative" medicine makes it more difficult for you to get the medical help you need.

This down-to-earth book lets patients take care of themselves. It also lets doctors who are not familiar with chronic mercury intoxication treat it. The book is a practical guide to getting well. Sections from the book include:

- Why worry about mercury poisoning?
- What mercury does to you – symptoms, laboratory test irregularities, diagnostic checklist.
- How to treat mercury poisoning easily with oral chelators.
- Dealing with other metals including copper, arsenic, lead, cadmium.
- Dietary and supplement guidelines.
- Balancing hormones during the recovery process.
- How to feel good while you are chelating the metals out.
- How heavy metals cause infections to thrive in the body.
- Politics and mercury.

This is the world's most authoritative, accurate book on mercury poisoning.

Paperback book, 8.5 x 11", 226 pages, $35

Hair Test Interpretation: Finding Hidden Toxicities

By Andrew Cutler, PhD

Hair tests are worth doing because a surprising number of people diagnosed with incurable chronic health conditions actually turn out to have a heavy metal problem; quite often, mercury poisoning. Heavy metal problems can be corrected. Hair testing allows the underlying problem to be identified – and the chronic health condition often disappears with proper detoxification.

Hair Test Interpretation: Finding Hidden Toxicities is a practical book that explains how to interpret **Doctor's Data, Inc.** and **Great Plains Laboratory** hair tests. A step-by-step discussion is provided, with figures to illustrate the process and make it easy. The book gives examples using actual hair test results from real people.

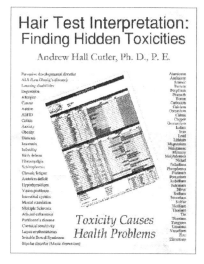

Hair Test Interpretation: Finding Hidden Toxicities

Andrew Hall Cutler, Ph. D., P. E.

Toxicity Causes Health Problems

Book • $35

One of the problems with hair testing is that both conventional and alternative health care providers do not know how to interpret these tests. Interpretation is not as simple as looking at the results and assuming that any mineral out of the reference range is a problem mineral.

Interpretation is complicated because heavy metal toxicity, especially mercury poisoning, interferes with mineral transport throughout the body. Ironically, if someone is mercury poisoned, hair test mercury is often low and other minerals may be elevated or take on unusual values. For example, mercury often causes retention of arsenic, antimony, tin, titanium, zirconium, and aluminum. An inexperienced health care provider may wrongfully assume that one of these other minerals is the culprit, when in reality mercury is the true toxicity.

"This new book of Andrew's is the definitive guide in the confusing world of heavy metal poisoning diagnosis and treatment. I'm a practicing physician, 20 years now, specializing in detoxification programs for treatment of resistant conditions. It was fairly difficult to diagnose these heavy metal conditions before I met Andrew Cutler and developed a close relationship with him while reading his books. In this book I found his usual painful attention to detail gave a solid framework for understanding the complexity of mercury toxicity as well as the less common exposures. You really couldn't ask for a better reference book on a subject most researchers and physicians are still fumbling in the dark about."
- Dr. Rick Marschall

So, as you can see, getting a hair test is only the first step. The second step is figuring out what the hair test means. Andrew Cutler, PhD, is a registered professional chemical engineer with years of experience in biochemical and healthcare research. This clear and concise book makes hair test interpretation easy, so that you know which toxicities are causing your health problems.

Paperback book, 8.5 x 11", 298 pages, $35

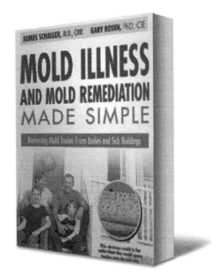

Book • $32.95

Mold Illness and Mold Remediation Made Simple: Removing Mold Toxins from Bodies and Sick Buildings

By James Schaller, M.D. and Gary Rosen, Ph.D.

Indoor mold toxins are much more dangerous and prevalent than most people realize. Visible mold in and around your house is far less dangerous than the mold you cannot see. Indoor mold toxicity, in addition to causing its own unique set of health problems and symptoms, also greatly contributes to the severity of most chronic illnesses.

In this book, a top physician and experienced contractor team up to help you quickly recover from indoor mold exposure. This book is easy to read with many color photographs and illustrations.

Dr. Schaller is a practicing physician in Florida who has written more than 15 books. He is one of the few physicians in the United States successfully treating mold toxin illness in children and adults.

Dr. Rosen is a biochemist with training under a Nobel Prize winning researcher at UCLA. He has written several books and is an expert in the mold remediation of homes. Dr. Rosen and his family are sensitive to mold toxins so he writes not only from professional experience, but also from personal experience.

Together, the two authors have certification in mold testing, mold remediation, and indoor environmental health. This book is one of the most complete on the subject, and includes discussion of the following topics:

- Potential mold problems encountered in new homes, schools, and jobs.
- Diagnosing mold illness.
- Mold as it relates to dryness and humidity.
- Mold toxins and cancer treatment.
- Mold toxins and relationships.
- Crawlspaces, basements, attics, home cleaning techniques, and vacuums.
- Training your eyes to discern indoor mold.
- Leptin and obesity.
- Appropriate/inappropriate air filters and cleaners.
- How to handle old, musty products, materials and books, and how to safely sterilize them.
- A description of various types of molds, images of them, and their relative toxicity.
- Blood testing and how to use it to find hidden health problems.
- The book is written in a friendly, casual tone that allows easy comprehension and information retention.

> "A concise, practical guide on dealing with mold toxins and their effects."
>
> **- Bryan Rosner**

Many people are affected by mold toxins. Are you? If you can find a smarter or clearer book on this subject, buy it!

Paperback book, 8.5 x 11", 140 pages, $32.95
Also available on our website as an eBook!

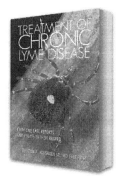

Treatment of Chronic Lyme Disease: 51 Case Reports and Essays In Their Regard

By Burton Waisbren Sr., MD, FACP, FIDSA

DON'T MISS THIS BOOK! A MUST-HAVE RESOURCE. What sets this Lyme disease book apart are the credentials of its author: he is not only a Fellow of the Infectious Diseases Society of America (IDSA), he is also one of its Founders! With 57+ years experience in medicine, Dr. Waisbren passionately argues for the validity of chronic Lyme disease and presents useful information about 51 cases of the disease which he has personally treated. His position is in stark contrast to that of the IDSA, which is a very powerful organization. **Quite possibly the most important book ever published on Lyme disease, as a result of the author's experience and credentials.**

Book • $24.95

Paperback book, 6x9", 169 pages, $24.95

Bartonella: Diagnosis and Treatment

By James Schaller, M.D.

2 Book Set • $99.95

As an addition to his growing collection of informative books, Dr. James Schaller penned this excellent 2-part volume on Bartonella, a Lyme disease co-infection. The set is an ideal complementary resource to his Babesia textbook (next page).

Bartonella infections occur throughout the entire world, in cities, suburbs, and rural locations. It is found in fleas, dust mites, ticks, lice, flies, cat and dog saliva, and insect feces.

This 2-book set provides advanced treatment strategies as well as detailed diagnostic criteria, with dozens of full-color illustrations and photographs.

Both books in this 2-part set are included with your order.

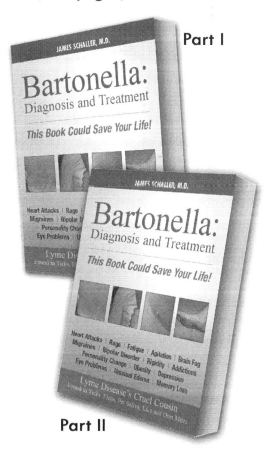

Part I

Part II

2 paperback books included, 7 x 10", 500 pages, $99.95

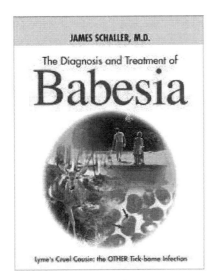

Book • $55

The Diagnosis and Treatment of Babesia: Lyme's Cruel Cousin – The Other Tick-Borne Infection

By James Schaller, M.D.

Do you or a loved one experience excess fatigue? Have you ever had unusually high fevers, chills, or sweats? You may have Babesia, a very common tick-borne infection. Babesia is often found with Lyme disease and, like all tick-borne infections, is rarely diagnosed and reported accurately.

The deer tick which carries Lyme disease and Babesia may be as small as a poppy seed and injects a painkiller, an antihistamine, and an anticoagulant to avoid detection. As a result, many people have Babesia and do not know it. Numerous forms of Babesia are carried by ticks. This book introduces patients and health care workers to the various species that infect humans and are not routinely tested for by sincere physicians.

Dr. Schaller, who practices medicine in Florida, first became interested in Babesia after one of his own children was infected with it. None of the elite pediatricians or child specialists could help. No one tested for Babesia or considered it a possible diagnosis. His child suffered from just two of these typical Babesia symptoms:

- Significant Fatigue
- Coughing
- Dizziness
- Trouble Thinking
- Fevers
- Memory Loss

- Chills
- Air Hunger
- Headache
- Sweats
- Unresponsiveness to Lyme Treatment

With 374 pages, this book is the most current and comprehensive book on Babesia in the English language. It reviews thousands of articles and presents the results of interviews with world experts on the subject. It offers you top information and broad treatment options, presented in a clear and simple manner. All treatments are explained thoroughly, including their possible side effects, drug interactions, various dosing strategies, pros/cons, and physician experiences.

"Once again Dr. Schaller has provided us with a much-needed and practical resource. This book gave me exactly what I was looking for."

- Thomas W., Patient

Finally, the book also addresses many other aspects of practical medical care often overlooked in this infection, such as treatment options for managing fatigue. Plainly stated, this book is a must-have for patients and health care providers who deal with Lyme disease and its co-infections. Dr. Schaller's many years in clinical practice give the book a practical angle that many other similar books lack. Don't miss this user-friendly resource!

Paperback book, 7 x 10", 374 pages, $55
Also available on our website as an eBook!

The Lyme Diet: Nutritional Strategies for Healing from Lyme Disease

By Nicola McFadzean, N.D.

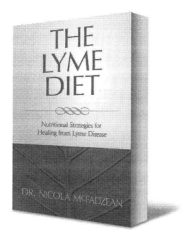

We know about antibiotics and herbs. But what is the right diet for Lyme sufferers? Now you can read about the experience of Dr. Nicola McFadzean, N.D., in treating Lyme patients using proper diet.

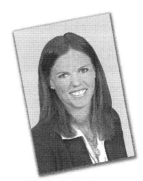

The author is a Naturopathic Doctor and graduate of Bastyr University in Seattle, Washington. She is currently in private practice at her clinic, RestorMedicine, located in San Diego, California.

Book • $24.95

Nicola McFadzean, N.D.

This book covers numerous topics (not just diet-related):

- Reducing and controlling inflammation
- Maximizing immune function via dietary choices
- Restoring the gut & regaining healthy digestion
- Detoxification with food
- Hormone imbalances
- Biofilms
- Kefir vs. yogurt vs. probiotics
- Candida, liver support, and much more!

Paperback book, 6x9", 214 Pages, $24.95
Also available as an eBook on our website!

The Stealth Killer: Is Oral Spirochetosis the Missing Link in the Dental & Heart Disease Labyrinth? *By William D. Nordquist, BS, DMD, MS*

Can oral spirochete infections cause heart attacks? In today's cosmopolitan urban population, more than 51 percent of those with root canal–treated teeth probably have infection at the apex of their root. Dr. Nordquist, an oral surgeon practicing in Southern California, believes that any source of bacteria with resulting chronic infection (including periodontal disease) in the mouth may potentially lead to heart disease and other systemic diseases. With more than 40 illustrations and x-ray reproductions, this book takes you behind the scenes in Dr. Nordquist's research laboratory, and provides many tips on dealing with Lyme-related dental problems. A breakthrough book in dentistry & infectious disease!

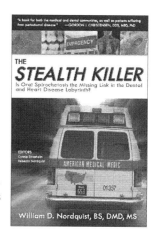

Paperback Book • $25.95

Paperback book, 6x9", 161 pages, $25.95

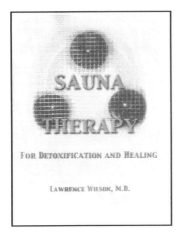

Book • $22.95

Sauna Therapy for Detoxification and Healing

By Lawrence Wilson, MD

This book provides a thorough yet articulate education on sauna therapy. It includes construction plans for a low-cost electric light sauna. The book is well referenced with an extensive bibliography.

Sauna therapy, especially with an electric light sauna, is one of the most powerful, safe and cost-effective methods of natural healing. It is especially important today due to extensive exposure to toxic metals and chemicals.

Fifteen chapters cover sauna benefits, physiological effects, protocols, cautions, healing reactions, and many other aspects of sauna therapy.

Dr. Wilson is an instructor of Biochemistry, Hair Mineral Analysis, Sauna Therapy and Jurisprudence at various colleges and universities including Yamuni Institute of the Healing Arts (Maurice, LA), University of Natural Medicine (Santa Fe, NM), Natural Healers Academy (Morristown, NJ), and Westbrook University (West Virginia). His books are used as textbooks at East-West School of Herbology and Ohio College of Natural Health. Go to www.LymeBook.com for free book excerpts!.

Paperback book, 8.5 x 11", 167 pages, $22.95

Physicians' Desk Reference (PDR) Books (opposing page)

Most people have heard of *Physicians' Desk Reference* (PDR) books because, for over 60 years, physicians and researchers have turned to PDR for the latest word on prescription drugs.

THOMSON ™

You may not know that Thomson Healthcare, publisher of PDR, offers PDR reference books not only

"I relied heavily on the PDRs during the research phase of writing my books. Without them, my projects would have greatly suffered."

- Bryan Rosner

for drugs, but also for herbal and nutritional supplements. No available books come even close to the amount of information provided in these PDRs—*PDR for Herbal Medicines* weighs 5 lbs and has over 1300 pages, and *PDR for Nutritional Supplements* weighs over 3 lbs and has more than 800 pages.

We carry all three PDRs. Although PDR books are typically used by physicians, we feel that these resources are also essential for people interested in or recovering from chronic disease. For the supplements, herbs, and drugs included in the books, you will find the following information: Pharmacology, description and method of action, available trade names and brands, indications and usage, research summaries, dosage options, history of use, pharmacokinetics, and much more! Worth the money for years of faithful use.

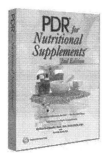

PDR for Nutritional Supplements *2nd Edition!*

This PDR focuses on the following types of supplements:

- Vitamins
- Minerals
- Amino acids
- Hormones
- Lipids
- Glyconutrients
- Probiotics
- Proteins
- Many more!

Book • $69.50

"In a part of the health field not known for its devotion to rigorous science, [this book] brings to the practitioner and the curious patient a wealth of hard facts."

- Roger Guillemin, M.D., Ph.D., Nobel Laureate in Physiology and Medicine

The book also suggests supplements that can help reduce prescription drug side effects, has full-color photographs of various popular commercial formulations (and contact information for the associated suppliers), and so much more! Become educated instead of guessing which supplements to take.

Hardcover book, 11 x 9.3", 800 pages, $69.50

PDR for Herbal Medicines *4th Edition!*

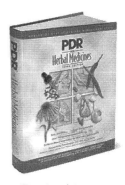

PDR for Herbal Medicines is very well organized and presents information on hundreds of common and uncommon herbs and herbal preparations. Indications and usage are examined with regard to homeopathy, Indian and Chinese medicine, and unproven (yet popular) applications.

In an area of healthcare so unstudied and vulnerable to hearsay and hype, this scientifically referenced book allows you to find out the real story behind the herbs lining the walls of your local health food store.

Use this reference before spending money on herbal products!

Book • $69.50

Hardcover book, 11 x 9.3", 1300 pages, $69.50

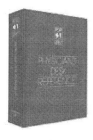

PDR for Prescription Drugs *Current Year's Edition!*

With more than 3,000 pages, this is the most comprehensive and respected book in the world on over 4,000 drugs. Drugs are indexed by both brand and generic name (in the same convenient index) and also by manufacturer and product category. This PDR provides usage information and warnings, drug interactions, plus a detailed, full-color directory with descriptions and cross references for the drugs. A new format allows dramatically improved readability and easier access to the information you need now.

Book • $99.50

Hardcover book, 12.5 x 9.5", 3533 pages, $99.50

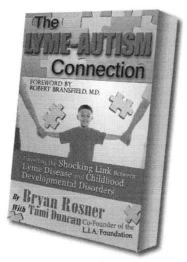

Book • $25.95

The Lyme-Autism Connection: Unveiling the Shocking Link Between Lyme Disease and Childhood Developmental Disorders
By Bryan Rosner & Tami Duncan

Did you know that Lyme disease may contribute to the onset of autism?

This book is an investigative report written by Bryan Rosner and Tami Duncan. Duncan is the co-founder of the *Lyme Induced Autism (LIA) Foundation*, and her son has an autism diagnosis.

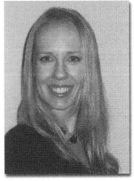

Tami Duncan, Co-Founder of the Lyme Induced Autism (LIA) Foundation

Awareness of the Lyme-autism connection is spreading rapidly, among both parents and practitioners. *Medical Hypothesis*, a scientific, peer-reviewed journal published by Elsevier, recently released an influential study entitled *The Association Between Tick-Borne Infections, Lyme Borreliosis and Autism Spectrum Disorders*. Here is an excerpt from the study:

> "Chronic infectious diseases, including tick-borne infections such as Borrelia burgdorferi, may have direct effects, promote other infections, and create a weakened, sensitized and immunologically vulnerable state during fetal development and infancy, leading to increased vulnerability for developing autism spectrum disorders. An association between Lyme disease and other tick-borne infections and autistic symptoms has been noted by numerous clinicians and parents."

—**Medical Hypothesis Journal.**
Article Authors: Robert C. Bransfield, M.D., Jeffrey S. Wulfman, M.D., William T. Harvey, M.D., Anju I. Usman, M.D.

Nationwide, 1 out of 150 children are diagnosed with Autism Spectrum Disorder (ASD), and the LIA Foundation has discovered that many of these children test positive for Lyme disease/Borrelia related complex—yet most children in this scenario never receive appropriate medical attention. This book answers many difficult questions: How can infants contract Lyme disease if autism begins before birth, precluding the opportunity for a tick bite? Is there a statistical correlation between the incidences of Lyme disease and autism worldwide? Do autistic children respond to Lyme disease treatment? What does the medical community say about this connection? Do the mothers of affected children exhibit symptoms? **Find out in this book.**

Paperback book, 6x9", 287 pages, $25.95

**Dietrich Klinghardt, M.D., Ph.D.
"Fundamental Teachings"
5-DVD Set**

Includes Disc Exclusively For Lyme Disease!

Dietrich Klinghardt, M.D., Ph.D. is a legendary healer known for discovering and refining many of the cutting-edge treatment protocols used for a variety of chronic health problems including Lyme disease, autism and mercury poisoning.

Now you can find out all about this doctor's treatment methods from the privacy of your own home! This 5-DVD set includes the following DVDs:

- **DISC 1**: The Five Levels of Healing and the Seven Factors
- **DISC 2**: Autonomic Response Testing and Demonstration
- **DISC 3**: Heavy Metal Toxicity and Neurotoxin Elimination / Electrosmog
- **DISC 4**: Lyme disease and Chronic Illness
- **DISC 5**: Psycho-Emotional Issues in Chronic Illness & Addressing Underlying Causes

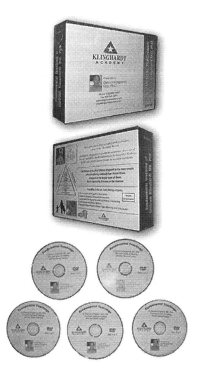

5-DVD Set • $125

Dr. Dietrich Klinghardt is one of the most important contributors to modern integrative treatment for Lyme disease and related medical conditions. This comprehensive DVD set is a must-have addition to your educational library.

5-DVD Set, $125

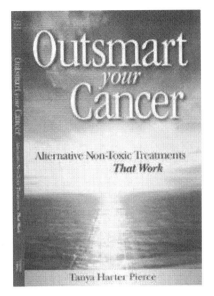

Book and Audio CD • $24.50

Outsmart Your Cancer: Alternative Non-Toxic Treatments That Work By Tanya Harter Pierce

Why BLUDGEON cancer to death with common conventional treatments that can be toxic and harmful to your entire body?

When you OUTSMART your cancer, only the cancer cells die — NOT your healthy cells! *OUTSMART YOUR CANCER: Alternative Non-Toxic Treatments That Work* is an easy guide to successful non-toxic treatments for cancer that you can obtain right now! In it, you will read real-life stories of people who have completely recovered from their advanced or late-stage lung cancer, breast cancer, prostate cancer, kidney cancer, brain cancer, childhood leukemia, and other types of cancer using effective non-toxic approaches.

Plus, *OUTSMART YOUR CANCER* is one of the few books in print today that gives a complete description of the amazing formula called "Protocel," which has produced incredible cancer recoveries over the past 20 years. **A supporting audio CD is included with this book.** Pricing = $19.95 book + $5.00 CD.

Paperback book, 6 x 9", 437 pages, with audio CD, $24.95

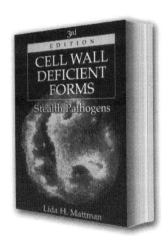

Hardcover Book • $169.95

Cell Wall Deficient Forms: Stealth Pathogens

By Lida Mattman, Ph.D.

This is one of the most influential infectious disease textbook of the century. Dr. Mattman, who earned a Ph.D. in immunology from Yale University, describes her discovery that a certain type of pathogen lacking a cell wall is the root cause of many of today's "incurable" and mysterious chronic diseases. Dr. Mattman's research is the foundation of our current understanding of Lyme disease, and her work led to many of the Lyme protocols used today (such as the Marshall Protocol, as well as modern LLMD antibiotic treatment strategy). Color illustrations and meticulously referenced breakthrough principles cover the pages of this book. A must have for all serious students of chronic, elusive infectious disease.

Hardcover book, 7.5 x 10.5", 416 pages, $169.95

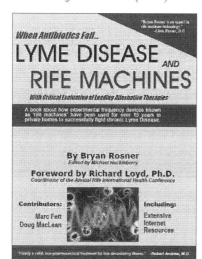

Book • $35

When Antibiotics Fail: Lyme Disease And Rife Machines, With Critical Evaluation Of Leading Alternative Therapies

By Bryan Rosner
Foreword by Richard Loyd, Ph.D.

There are enough books and websites about what Lyme disease is and which ticks carry it. But there is very little useful information for people who actually have a case of Lyme disease that is not responding to conventional antibiotic treatment. Lyme disease sufferers need to know their options, not how to identify a tick.

This book describes how experimental electromagnetic frequency devices known as rife machines have been used for over 15 years in private homes to fight Lyme disease. Also included are evaluations of more than 25 conventional and alternative Lyme disease therapies, including:

- Homeopathy
- IV and oral antibiotics
- Mercury detox.
- Hyperthermia / saunas
- Ozone and oxygen
- Samento®
- Colloidal Silver
- Bacterial die-off detox.

- Colostrum
- Magnesium supplementation
- Hyperbaric oxygen chamber (HBOC)
- ICHT Italian treatment
- Non-pharmaceutical antibiotics
- Exercise, diet and candida protocols
- Cyst-targeting antibiotics
- The Marshall Protocol®

Many Lyme disease sufferers have heard of rife machines, some have used them. But until now, there has not been a concise and organized source to explain how and why they have been used by Lyme patients. In fact, this is the first book ever published on this important topic.

The Foreword for the book is by Richard Loyd, Ph.D., coordinator of the annual Rife International Health Conference. The book takes a practical, down-to-earth approach which allows you to learn about*:

> "This book provides life-saving insights for Lyme disease patients."
>
> **- Richard Loyd, Ph.D.**

- Antibiotic treatment problems and shortcomings—why some people choose to use rife machines after other therapies fail.
- Hypothetical treatment schedules and sessions, based on the author's experience.
- The experimental machines with the longest track record: High Power Magnetic Pulser, EMEM Machine, Coil Machine, and AC Contact Machine.
- Explanation of the "herx reaction" and why it may indicate progress.
- The intriguing story that led to the use of rife machines to fight Lyme disease 20 years ago.
- Antibiotic categories and classifications, with pros and cons of each type of drug.
- Visit our website to read FREE EXCERPTS from the book!

Disclaimer: *Your treatment decisions must be made under the care of a licensed physician. Rife machines are not FDA approved and the FDA has not reviewed or approved of these books. The author is a layperson, not a doctor, and much of the content of these books is a statement of opinion based on the author's personal experience and research.*

Paperback book, 8.5 x 11", 203 pages, $35

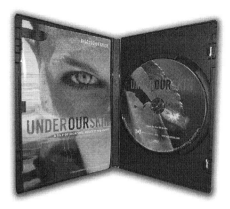

**Under Our Skin:
Lyme Disease Documentary
Film**

A gripping tale of microbes, medicine & money, UNDER OUR SKIN exposes the hidden story of Lyme disease, one of the most serious and controversial epidemics of our time. Each year, thousands go undiagnosed or misdiagnosed, often told that their symptoms are all in their head.

DVD • $34.95

Following the stories of patients and physicians fighting for their lives and livelihoods, the film brings into focus a haunting picture of the health care system and a medical establishment all too willing to put profits ahead of patients.

Bonus Features: 32-page discussion guidebook, one hour of bonus footage, director's commentary, and much more! <u>FOR HOME USE ONLY</u>

DVD with bonus features, 104 minutes, $34.95 *MUST SEE!*

Ordering is Easy!

Phone: **Toll Free (866) 476-7637**
Online: **www.LymeBook.com**

Detailed product information and secure online ordering is available on our website. Bulk orders to bookstores, health food stores, or Lyme disease support groups – call us for wholesale terms.

Do you have a book inside you? Submit your book proposal online at: www.lymebook.com/submit-book-proposal.

Join Lyme Community Forums at: www.lymecommunity.com.

Get paid to help us place our books in your local health food store. Learn more: www.lymebook.com/local-store-offer.

DISCLAIMER

This disclaimer is in reference to all books, DVDs, websites, flyers, and catalogs published by Bryan Rosner, DBA BioMed Publishing Group.

Our materials are for informational and educational purposes only. They are not intended to prevent, diagnose, treat, or cure disease. Some of the treatments described are not FDA-Approved. Bryan Rosner is a layperson, not a medical professional, and he is not qualified to dispense medical advice.

These books and DVDs are not intended to substitute for professional medical care. Do not postpone receiving care from a licensed physician. Please read our full disclaimer online at: www.lymebook.com/homepage-disclaimer.pdf.

Made in the USA
Charleston, SC
21 March 2013